Mission Statement

My mission is to raise human consciousness and change all systems.

My vision is clean air, water, soil, and equitable systems
for all mankind... in my lifetime.

- Troy Casey

#RIPPEDAT50
A JOURNEY TO SELF LOVE

"#RIPPEDAT50 is a fascinating journey into holistic health;
a concise guide to fulfilling your potential at any age."

Dorian Yates, 6X Mr. Olympia turned Truth-Seeker.

TROY CASEY

FOREWORD BY PAUL CHEK

#RIPPEDAT50: A Journey to Self Love

Troy Casey, Sedona, AZ,
USA

CertifiedHealthNut.com
Instagram: @certifiedhealthnut
Twitter: @mrhealthnut
Facebook: Certified Health Nut

ISBN: 978-1-7344073-0-3 (hardcover)
ISBN: 978-1-7344073-2-7 (paperback)
ISBN: 978-1-7344073-1-0 (digital)

Praise for #RIPPEDAT50 and Troy Casey

"The advice that the 'seats of power' give on growing old is to sit on your ass, get real fat, sedate the pain, and die on your back. Troy and I say there's a different way. It's a sin not to grin, so take off your shoes, move your body and BE HAPPY!"

Mick Dodge, the "Barefoot Sensei,"
TV personality, Rainforest Dweller

"Troy brings the primal man back in modern society, with greater balance and wisdom than I've seen anyone embody. The result is a no BS, highly ALIVE way of being, breathing, and LIVING. If you want to become an unstoppable force of nature with limitless energy—he is your guy."

"Ryno" Ryan Hughes,
Motocross Champion of the World!

"Told with authenticity, Troy's book isn't about vanity, it's about your total health, wellbeing and real living. Read it and practice!"

Michael Beckwith, Best-Selling Author and Founder of
Agape International Spiritual Center in Beverly Hills, CA

"As someone behind $2 billion in infomercial sales, I know a thing or two about selling and charisma. What I love about Troy is how he helps you tap into the limitless, youthful energy inside your body—to unlock your own natural inspiration, charisma, and power. He's certainly *sold* me!"

Forbes Riley, Billionaire Business Strategist,
Celebrity TV Host, Infomercial Queen

"Troy combines the wisdom of and mastery of a man who's been in the game for decades. Every sentence proceeds from knowing and the compassion to see others succeed."

**Elliott Hulse, Strongman, Author,
and Strength Coach to millions of men worldwide**

"Troy has combined all the elements needed to create a LIFE of wellness. Thank you, Troy, for your wisdom and your journey."

**Mariel Hemingway,
American Actress, Author, and Health Icon**

"Troy Casey is a living breathing Being that embodies growth. His approach and practice of Eastern Energetics and Modern Athletics create a Timeless Physique. Nutrients both Organic and Spiritual feed His Journey. Strap in. The Ride is Waiting for all who Need More True Life."

**Rudy Reyes, former active duty US Marine,
Fitness and Martial Arts Mentor, Speaker, and Partner of Force
Blue**

"Troy Casey is a radical person. His book #RIPPEDAT50 will help you shatter the confines of "normal" health and quality of life so you can look and feel rejuvenated. To get radical results you need a radical guide. In #RIPPEDAT50 Troy is that guide that'll help you unapologetically march right past the norms of mediocrity right into the radical health, energy, and quality of life you've been dreaming of."

**JP Sears, American Life Coach,
Author and Internet Comedian**

"Troy Casey is filled with knowledge and health hacks that we all need. Accessible and super smart; I highly recommend his new book for those of us that see age as a blessing and who are fifty plus as it's time to bring our best selves to all that we are and do."

Carrie Anne Moss, Canadian Actress and founder of Annapurna Living, a lifestyle brand designed to empower women through mindfulness, meditation & devotion

---

"Troy has taught me a lot... I was reluctant at first to try some of his certified nutty routines, but they always seem to work. And we laughed in the process which as we all know is the best medicine. Thanks Troy!"

Simon Rex, American Actor, rapper, comedian, and model

"A lot of people talk about change or getting healthy, but Troy Casey has made it his life's work to spread the message of healthy food and an active lifestyle to as many people as possible. As the Certified Health Nut, Troy Casey is on a one-man mission to help individuals navigate the sometimes confusing road to health, mental fitness and spiritual wellbeing. Even if you may never reach all your own #RIPPEDAT50 goals, joining the Certified Health Nut on this healing journey is one you can't afford to miss."

Dave Murphy, writer, activist, and founder of Food Democracy Now!

Foreword

L IFE HAS CHANGED for all of us in the past 100 years. The advancements made in electronics and information technologies, have increased our pace of life, and left us in a perpetual rush, losing our roots, losing our connections to the earth and each other.

We are being bombarded by chemicals and junk food, and we have fallen for the myth of consumerism. We are experiencing a deep emptiness from losing vital connections to family, friends, and even ourselves. Artificial intelligence is being used to create the illusion of efficiency, while also being used to manipulate you into believing and doing things that are not in your best interest; things that don't support the planet, and direct massive profits into the hands of the few, sadly, the few that only seem to care about profits, not people or the planet.

In the 35 years of my own career in holistic health, corrective, and high-performance exercise and spiritual development, I have seen every kind of injury or illness that people can unintentionally bring upon themselves simply by being unaware of "how to live." My work as an educator, therapist, and holistic lifestyle coach has taken me around the world many, many times, allowing me to see the ongoing degeneration of many cultures, all for the same reasons that Troy Casey beautifully addresses in this book, #RIPPEDAT50.

As an educator and a therapist, I interact with a wide variety of people, from those who want someone to "fix" them, to those simply dabbling in the current health fad, and to those who have a genuine passion for health, and an interest in the wellbeing of the planet and nature at large. Troy Casey is a man bursting with passion for health, the well-being of the people, and the planet. He has been a student of mine for many years, and in that time, I've watched him engage his health, fitness, relationships, parenting, and global activism, more fully than anyone I know. To this day, I wear his "Certified Health Nut" t-shirts with pride.

Troy has studied, applied, lived, and shared the six foundation principles I teach through the C.H.E.K Institute's Holistic Lifestyle Coaching program, and he beautifully shares his journey and his knowledge of the principles of nutrition, hydration, sleep, breathing, thinking, and movement in #RIPPEDAT50.

#RIPPEDAT50 is an exciting exploration into Troy's life and will inspire you to become healthier, more vital, more honest, and more open with yourself and with others. I hope you enjoy becoming whole with Troy as much as I do each day!

Love and chi,

Paul Chek, H.H.P.
Founder, C.H.E.K Institute
Founder, PPS Success Mastery

Gratitude

FOR THE LOVERS, artists, fire-starters, and inspirational motivators!

#1 the Ineffable Great Spirit.

My beautiful supportive wife Uri Lee and my children Troy and Athena, who support me with the nourishment of love.

My ancestors.

My step-father who raised me.

My mother, Ann Philips.

My biological father, James Casey.

My grandmother, Marguerite Yemens, and grandfather, Charlie Yemens. My Grandfather James Casey and Grandmother Eileen Casey.

Paul Chek and all the CHEK Practitioners worldwide who hold the bar high for holistic health, Paul Lubicz, Chaba Lucas, Papa Joe (RIP) and the Maori Healers, Atarangi Muru, Terence Muru, and Dr. Mercola, for forwarding health consciousness in the media.

Real Estate Mogul, Brian Culhane.

Amazon John Easterling, Mike Baiochhi, Jonas Koffler, Gary Rhodes, Elliot Hulse, Scott Petersen, Dr. Richard Schultz, Mariel Hemingway, Bobby Williams, Alex Hill, Rudy Reyes, Andrew Eckert, Ra of Earth, Carolina Rocha, Curtis Guild, David Sandoval, Amy Venner, Baron Baptiste, Bryan Kest, Andy Mills, Caroline Gaskin, and the Holistic Justice League of wellness entrepreneurs that have joined me in business to forward these ideas to the popular culture.

Legendary Barefoot Sensei, Mick Dodge.

Visionaries who forwarded the ideas of peace and harmony by any means necessary: Rudolf Steiner, Buckminster Fuller, Nikola Tesla, Paramahansa Yogananda and S.N. Goenka, Swami Sachasananda (whom my father James studied with at the Integral Yoga Institute), Malcolm X, Nelson Mandela, Viktor Frankl, MLK, Mahatma Gandhi.

Joe Rogan, JP Sears, Bob Proctor, Les Brown, Mark Victor Hansen, John Assaraf, Dr. Joe Dispenza.

The hip hop community that gave me an avenue to channel my angst and a way to focus my artistic creativity into something positive, taking the mind-over-matter and rags-to-riches principles to a whole other level of motivation and inspiration. The Def Jam camp of the late 80's, Rick Rubin, Russell Simmons, RUN DMC, Beastie boys, LL Cool J, the West Coast all stars: NWA, Digital Underground, Tupac, Freestyle Fellowship, Pharcyde, and, of course, the next wave of NYC flavor: Wu Tang Clan, especially the Old Dirty Bastard (RIP), who lived without filters, Biggie and the teacher KRS One (still #1), Gucci Mane and Kodak Black for taking the street mentality into full-blown artistic creativity.

Arnold Schwarzenegger & Kron Gracie and the Gracie Brazilian Jiu Jitsu family legacy. Jack LaLanne, the first Certified Health Nut.

Refugio Alti Plano, Shamanic Healing Center, Peru, where I received powerful healing and visions for the path I AM on now.

Elisa Vargas Fernandez from the village of San Francisco de Yarinacocha, Pucallpa, Ucayali, Peru, and all the Shipibo Indians who taught me about Ayahuasca and Amazonian plant medicines.

The artists of the world who inspired me to just do it and create something out of nothing: Andy Warhol, Shepard Fairey, Banksy, Alex Grey, Salvador Dali, David LaChapelle, Justin BUA, Gianni Versace.

And all the starving artists who dedicate their lives to utilizing art to affect and shift consciousness.

Preface

"If you are looking for confirmation bias, look in the scientific literature, because it is always there. If you are looking for actual results, then look in the mirror."

Dr. Shawn Baker

HI FRIEND. YOU don't know me, so before you start reading this book, I thought I'd take a minute to set some expectations. I'd like for us to get off on the right foot.

If you picked up this book because of its cover, you might think #RIPPEDAT50 is a diet book. After all, any dude my age with six-pack abs must really be watching what he eats, right?

Well, yes and no. Yes, I am very particular about what I put into my body. But no...this is no diet book.

If I tell you that my intention in writing this book is to elevate your spirit and help you reclaim your divinity, you might think #RIPPEDAT50 is about religion. Again, you'd be wrong.

And if I told you not to shit in your proverbial spoon and shove it in your mouth you might think, "What the fuck did he just say?"

Spoiler alert – this book contains some strong language, some adult situations, and some out-of-the-mainstream ideas. (Oh shit, was I supposed to say, "spoiler alert" before I said "fuck?" Sorry!)

Anyway, now you've been warned. So, are you cool with some non-conventional thinking and the occasional four-letter word? If not, now's the time to turn back. Maybe you can even get your money back for the book.

But if you decide to proceed, I predict this book will change your life. If you're looking to get ripped, this book will put you well on your way. It's packed with a ton of knowledge and actionable information you can use to radically change your physique. I did it and so can you!

But I hope you'll come away from this book with much more than that. #RIPPEDAT50 is about living life optimally. It is about finding balance in mind, body, and spirit. #RIPPEDAT50 is about the journey to self love.

Let's get this out in the open: like Neo in the Matrix, I am here to tell you that most of the people on this planet spend their days in a prison of their own minds. They are controlled by powerful and nefarious forces whose goal is to enrich themselves at any cost. But at the end of the day, I can't really tell you any of that. I had to experience it for myself and so do you.

My hope is that this book will inspire you to do some mirror gazing of your own. I hope you can get right with yourself, recognize those things you need to work on and use the tools you have been endowed with to reach your goals.

So what I've done is this: I've poured my heart out in these pages. I've told my story as honestly as I know how, warts and all. I've distilled what I've learned in my personal journal down into 9 Pillars, and I've given you some concrete steps you can take to improve each pillar of your life.

You've been given a priceless machine, my friend! Your mind, your body, and your soul are yours. The ineffable spirit gifted you a Ferrari, and when it is tuned up and running the way it was built to run, you won't believe how good it feels to be behind the wheel!

But high-end machines are complex. They need to be maintained and cared for. You need to love yourself and take care of yourself because you are one of a kind. You are precious and valuable beyond compare. In some ways, you can use #RIPPEDAT50 like a mainte-nance manual.

I treated my engine like shit for years! I was reckless and wild and, but for the grace of God, I might be splayed out in a ditch somewhere, crushed and twisted beyond recognition.

But I found my purpose and my vision. I've freed myself from the prison of my own mind. I've found gratitude, and love, and forgiveness, and it is wonderful. I drank the plant medicine. I went on spiritual ventures. I healed my body and my mind.

The truth is, I want to change the world. Crazy, right? Or is it?

#RIPPEDAT50 is not about converting you to my way of thinking. It doesn't have a political agenda. It doesn't preach or point the finger. I am not trying to sell you anything, and I am not looking for followers.

Truth be told, I think our species stands on the blade of a knife, and the horrors committed on this planet every day could make you believe that there is hell on earth. But I've seen visions and I know that humanity makes it. My heart is bursting with hope.

If we're going to solve our problems, we need clarity. All knowledge is knowledge of self. We have to stand naked in front of the mirror – literally and figuratively – and be honest with ourselves. #RIPPEDAT50 is not about me and my physique.

It's about standing naked in front of the mirror and being honest. And that's not easy. But I've done the best I can. This book is my story, as best as I can tell it. I hope you like it.

I am not going to tell you how to read this book. You might read it cover to cover in one sitting. Then again, you might just pick it up with your morning coffee like an oracle, turn to a random page, and find a bit of wisdom that you can incorporate in your life. It's up to you. But whatever you do, my solemn advice is this: Take everything in this book with a grain of salt, a pinch of humor, and the seriousness of death, as if your life depended on it.

And be open to miracles.

Troy Casey, H.H.P.
C.H.E.K. Practitioner
International Speaker
Founder, Certified Health Nut

Contents

LEGACY

CHAPTER ONE

misnomer – wrong or inaccurate name or designation.

*"Either define the moment
or the moment will define you."*

Walt Whitman

I GUESS YOU COULD say I had a bad case of the "fuckits." Everyone was back in Milan for men's fashion week, and we all checked into the same hotel. Things were getting out of hand. Anything less would have been unfashionable.

It was the Summer of '96, and I was running for Mayor of Drunksville. A hard-core campaigner, my poll numbers were good, but the competition was stiff. I wasn't the only oversexed, strung-out, alcoholic male model in Milan, but I *was* going to be the most outrageous. This was my year! These Italians always brought out the best in me. Or the worst, depending on your point of view.

A dozen or so of us were on our way to a "Dancing for Dollars" party in Como, which, really, was a bit of a misnomer. We didn't actually have to dance. Our heroin-chic bodies and dead-on-the-inside eyes were worth the price of admission. But it had a catchy name and it stuck. I really hated these things, yet I never seemed to miss one. Go figure.

Mobbed-up owners wanted beautiful people in their clubs. People would stand in line and pay sinful cover fees just to be seen with us. Well...mostly they wanted the female models, but guys were part of the package.

Mob "runners" would roll into our hotel with booze and drugs. There was a party up in the mountains. Or down by the sea. Or who cares where. Who wants to go? Free drinks all night. I was all in! We'd jump on a train and party our asses off as we zipped across the Italian countryside. The drinks flowed freely. Coke piled up like drifts of snow blown down from the Alps. And for those of us with a taste for something more, heroin was plentiful and easy to pick up at any station along the way.

I bought a balloon at Milano Centrale, and by the time we rolled into Como, I had my head in the right place. Well, right place if my goal was to take a wrecking ball to this fucked-up industry and my place in it. So yeah...I was in the proper state of mind.

The club was one of those places where aspiring Cosa Nostra bosses rolled up in Ferraris with their wannabe-model girlfriends. The cover fee was – literally and figuratively – a crime, but a mere pittance for the honor of being in the room with Versace models.

I unloaded the rest of my ecstasy in under an hour and had a wad of cash in my front pocket that made me look like I was really happy to be there.

"What are you up to tonight?"

"Dancing for Dollars down in Genoa. Wanna come?"

I usually took a table in a dark corner and had bottle service all night. There was always a contingent of a half-dozen women who wanted to brag to their girlfriends about fucking a Versace model, and I was happy to oblige. Sometimes it was a quickie in the bathroom stall or splayed on the still-warm hood of a Maserati, but in this anything-goes club, BJs under the table were très chic.

When "Gangsta's Paradise" started blaring over the sound system, I was on the dance floor. Ecstasy was surging through my system, releasing massive amounts of serotonin. My mind was awash in a chemical stew of alcohol and neurotransmitters that brought both, an overwhelming sense of oneness with the world, and a pervasive feeling of fuckit.

Stumbling out of the place at 6:30 am, I fell across the hood of a '96 Lamborghini inconveniently parked at the curb. That set everybody off. It was the stumble of the season. A comedic gem. A goddamn riot of hilarity!

I bounced up laughing and got all tangled up with the car's owner. Or, more likely, the owner's shitty son. I could tell right away he liked to pump iron and flex in front of full-length mirrors.

"You fell on my car," he said, not smiling.

"Watch where you park that thing! You could hurt someone." I laughed and tried to get away, but he wasn't having it.

"You're right. I *could* hurt someone." He tried to look tough but was a little too short and fat to pull it off. I got my Ph.D. in smartass, and a softball like that across the fat part of the plate was just too much to resist. So I teed off.

"Based on your obviously low IQ," I said holding my fingers up to his face in a camera gesture, "coupled with your Cro-Magnon features, I'd say you hurt a lot of people already. Not the least of which, probably, your mamma."

He stood there with a stupid look on his face, the tiny gears in his brain grinding away, trying to comprehend what I'd just said. I used the pause to dash away, running and howling with laughter down the steps and across the street to the station where I hopped on the train just as the doors were closing. I raised my middle finger in a West Coast salute as the train pulled out of the station, leaving the Cro-Magnon and his tribe of greaseballs fuming on the platform.

At least that is the fantasy that flitted through my drug-addled brain. The reality was a bit messier. I took two steps, tripped on a curb, and went down on my face. Cro and the boys proceeded to kick the shit out of me and, based on the amount of laughter and high-fives they gave each other, they were having a pretty good time doing it.

By the time we got back to Milan, it was already hot as hell. I had fallen behind in my drinking on the train ride back – as I was literally and figuratively licking my wounds from the ass-kicking. Lack of alcohol, more than anything, was making me queasy.

"Are you okay, Troy?" asked Marco with a concerned look on his face.

I puked into a trashcan, breathing deeply the acrid smells of stomach acid, churros, oysters, and a cigar butt.

"Yeah, I'm okay," I said, wiping my mouth. "I just need a drink."

"Me too," said Kristoff as the three of us headed across the plaza under the Duomo.

The Duomo di Milano is the third biggest church in Europe. People travel from all around the world just to see it, but it's not my cup of tea. The statues seemed to stare down at me with disgust. I've heard stories, and not all those "saints" were what they're cracked up to be either, so the disgust was mutual.

The bar was officially closed, but we knew the bartender and got him laid from time to time. So he set us up.

"Troy, you should come to Ellio's with us today." "No thanks."

Ellio was a major player in the Italian fashion industry and had the ability to make or break a career. He was also a major perv and someone I wanted to stay as far away from as possible.

"He likes you," said Stephan with a knowing look.

"Not interested," I said as I finished a beer and helped myself to a refill.

"Jesus, Troy," Marco said, shaking his head. "You've gotta play this game better."

"I don't wanna play."

"Then why are you even here?"

"For the drinks, of course." I downed another pint to underscore the point. "You're drinking more than when I last saw you," Marco says.

"Thanks for noticing. I've been working hard at it."

"Ellio got me on the new Armani campaign," Stephan bragged. "And all you had to do was suck his dick," teased Kristoff.

"I *wish* it was that easy," Stephan replied. "But not half as gross as that fat pig you had to do to get the Gucci shoot."

"Touché." They toasted.

I met Ellio seven years before. It was 1989, and I was in Milan for the first time. I'd only been modeling for six months and had already scored a Versace ad. I was starting to believe all the beautiful lies my manager was telling me, except in my version my cock was even bigger.

Physically, Ellio was about as far from a male model as one could be. He was short and fat with a face not even a mother could love, and a personality to match. The fact that his name was synonymous with male modeling in Milan was not so much cruel irony as coldblooded revenge. He surrounded himself with beautiful boys and told them such lies! He took so much pleasure building them up before ruining them that I had him pegged as a sociopath from the moment I shook his hand.

"So...I hear you're going to be the next big thing," he said. I didn't like the way he put his hand on my chest.

"We'll see," I said. What a cocky little shit I was.

"With my help...there is no doubt!" He started to put his hand on my ass, but I stepped forward and pretended to ignore him.

"Quite a view you've got here," I said. The city stretched out in every direction from his balcony. There were also a couple dozen male models in Speedos lounging around the pool below. I could see his reflection in the glass when he smiled and responded, "Yes, quite a view."

He was an octopus with years of groping experience. I was a rookie who didn't want to alienate a potential ally but also couldn't stand being taken advantage of. Gasoline meet fire. It took everything I had not to smash his ugly face with the Ketel One bottle I was getting to know pretty well.

After being rebuffed for 10 minutes or so, Ellio suddenly remembered a call he had to make and waddled out of the room. I hadn't even poured another drink before his recruiters swooped in.

"Did you hear about Joel?" one of them said to the other, loud enough so that I could hear. "Ellio got him Calvin Klein."

"Shut up!"

Ellio was nothing if not obnoxiously heavy-handed. There was barely a space in the room that didn't feature him with some famous model, celebrity, tastemaker, billionaire, or – my personal favorite – Third World strongman. The 4 x 6 framed glossy of him and Muammar Gaddafi in the bathroom really piqued my interest. But then again, maybe it was Santana. I could never tell the two apart.

The recruiters talked about how rich Ellio was. How many careers he helped and how many careers he destroyed. How big his cock was. Seriously! One of them actually said something about his 10-inch eggplant. He'd have to take acting lessons for another 10 years to sell that line.

What did Ellio have on these poor kids that put them under his thumb? Or did they really think he'd put them on the map? At any rate, they did his bragging for him while slowly mixing their drinks, then sauntered away just as he reappeared.

"You're going places, Troy," he said, throwing his fat arm over my shoulder.

My amygdala fired. Epinephrine and adrenaline flooded my system. My hypothalamus prepared my body for violent muscular reaction. The hairs stood up on the back of my neck. Classic fight-or-flight response.

Unfortunately, this wasn't the first creepy old man (or woman) to put their hands on me.

I dropped my glass, which shattered into a million pieces on his immaculate marble floor. Just then, a bronze skinned, muscle-bound German cyborg skittered up barefoot and soon it was a bloody mess.

I used the chaos of the moment to make a quick escape. Later, I heard what a foul mood that put Ellio in and saw the purple welt he left on Derrick's ass for letting me get away so soon.

Over the next few years, he tried to lure me back into his web, but I managed (mostly) to steer clear. Ellio is the kind of enemy who, if he captured you, would nurse you back to health before he began torturing you. I knew he had nothing but terrible plans for me, yet he was always all smiles when we met.

"When are you going to come to me, Troy? I could help you," he'd say, always trying to lay his sausage-like fingers on my thigh or stick a pinkie up my bunghole.

He took particular pleasure in turning straight men into his boy toys, and I think I became an obsession of his. The one who got away. I lost more gigs than I can count, thanks to him. He foiled my plans, cut off my options and routes of escape. A real bastard.

I've heard all the apologist arguments. "Everybody's kinda gay." No. Not really.

We made our way back to the hotel at about noon. Stephan and Marco freshened up and headed over to Ellio's for a Caligula revival. I spent the afternoon sucking down Tylenol and Morettis and wondering if I had a fractured rib. At one point I actually thought about going to the hospital, but I didn't really want to spend money on doctors, so I walked over to the train station and scored another balloon of heroin.

By 8:00, I was back to my old self as we headed out to the Versace Fashion Show. The big buzz was that Gianni Versace had personally convinced Tupac Shakur to walk his show. For a lot of the guys, it was sour grapes and racist bullshit, but for me it was the first time in a long time I was actually excited about fashion week. I am a huge hip hop fan, and "Me Against the World" was becoming the soundtrack to my life.

I didn't have an invite to Versace's mansion that night to watch live, but they were broadcasting it on huge screens in Piazza del Duomo, so we hung out with the crowds. Watching Tupac walk the runway that night was beautiful. Seeing him perform "California Love" with Dr. Dre was transcendent. Of course, the ecstasy helped, but Tupac radiated a life force that was undeniable. Lightning in a bottle. It was electrifying.

Within three months, he'd be dead, and the world would lose a beautiful artist forever. Within a year, Gianni Versace would be murdered in Miami Beach. But on that summer night in 1996, life and art and fashion and music exploded out of Milan.

We heard Tupac was going to be at Club Hollywood for the after party, and I made it my mission to get in.

If you believe in such things, I suppose I am genetically blessed. Ever since I can remember, my looks have provoked strong reactions. Older kids wanted to be me. Girls...and then women...wanted to be *with* me. Whatever.

There are a lot of pretty people who never get a Versace ad. I got four of them. My looks helped, but I think the reason I made it so far was my ability to talk my way into – or out of – almost any situation. The gift of gab. A good conversationalist. The ability to BS. Call it what you will, I had it, and (mostly) used it to my advantage.

Of course, my smart mouth was also the cause of many of my life's most epic failures and painful beatings.

I talked my way into the place, and within 30 minutes I had BS'd my way right up to Tupac's table. He was holding court with Kidada Jones at his side and his bodyguards behind him. Nobody was going to fuck with Tupac that night.

He was from Oakland, and I grew up in Marin County, so we had some common ground. I told him how much I loved his music and thought he should be a movie star. He liked the sound of that. I had heard he was friends with Jada Pinkett Smith, and we talked about her for a while.

"I loved her in Menace II Society," I told him. "You should do a movie with her."

That lit him up but pissed Kidada off. She excused herself. He talked about changing his name to Makaveli. He had read Machiavelli's "The Prince" in prison and said it changed his life.

Before long, he was whisked away, talking to Donatella Versace. The next thing I knew, he was in the DJ booth doing an impromptu performance of "California Love." The place erupted.

California knows how to party In the city of L.A.
In the city of good ol' Watts
In the city, the city of Compton
We keep it rockin', we keep it rockin'

The next few days were a blur. Tupac set the fashion world on fire. July in Milan was a steamy, sexy party, and I was a hot mess.

Everyone was at Tutti Frutti for the Dolce & Gabbana party. Or was it Moschino? I can't remember. Anyway, it had been four days since the Versace show, and I don't think I'd slept since. I used heroin, cocaine, and ecstasy like a stonemason uses mortar. Applied expertly and in just the right amounts, they cemented each liquid moment to the next, allowing me to build an ever-higher wall of alcohol around myself.

The place was crowded, and I needed to make a grand entrance. So I stripped off all my clothes and did a backflip into the pool.

I got a smattering of applause, but not what I'd hoped for. Security didn't think it was funny at all. They dragged me out of the pool and told me to get the hell out of there.

"Come on, guys," I said. "Look around. Everybody's having a good time." I pointed to a couple obviously having sex under a beach towel. "Those two are having a *real* good time."

"You're making a scene."

"She's making a scene," I say, pointing to a young Calvin Klein model lying topless nearby. "And *he's* making a spectacle." An Austrian model walked by in a Speedo so tight I could tell he'd been circumcised. "What am I doing that is bothering anybody?"

"You can't do backflips in the pool."

"I didn't see the sign," I say. "Now I've been warned."

I walked away and they didn't follow. Damn! Where's the spectacle in that. I walked to the other side of the pool, and then whistled loudly.

The room went quiet, and the security guards scowled.

I turned dramatically, as if going for the gold. I lined up, checked my distance. Hands at my side, then up at 90 degrees. The crowd waited breathlessly.

I did another backflip into the pool. In my mind, it was beautiful and graceful, and I slipped into the water without so much as a ripple. Logically, I know it could not have been so pretty. I could barely walk, let alone perform gold-medal dives. But in my mind's eye, it was perfect.

That got the response I wanted! People were whistling and cheering as the guards dragged me out of the pool again. The couple that was having sex had finished and was now smoking cigarettes. They were positively glowing and smiled as I staggered past. I can't help but believe my dive put the cherry on top of their orgasm.

I got a call from my manager the next morning asking me to come see him. He was pissed.

"What the hell, Troy! You can't act like that?" "Sorry, mom," I said, putting my feet up on his desk. "What are you trying to prove?"

I shrugged my shoulders. I probably couldn't have articulated it anyway. "You can't act like that!"

"Why not? This whole industry is about who can be the most outrageous. 'Look at me, everybody! I haven't eaten a meal in 3 ½ years, and I could literally starve to death.

Aren't I beautiful?'"

He shook his head, lit a cigarette, and blew smoke dramatically. "Troy, I am gonna have to let you go."

"Jesus Christ, Don. You could have just told me that on the phone instead of making me come all the way down to this shithole of an office." I got up and made my way to the door. "Saves me the trouble of firing you. I have a better offer, and this takes away any guilt I might have felt."

I had a show in four hours, but I needed a drink. I ducked into a bar across the street where, for once, I actually paid for the alcohol. This didn't slow me down for one second.

By the time I got backstage, I was a hot mess. I hadn't slept or showered in days, and my eyes were bloodshot. My jeans were ripped and filthy, and I had a four-day beard and was dripping with sweat.

"Hey, is that Greg Louganis," sneered Paul as I stumbled in. He and Mathew held up judges' scorecards: 3.2 and 2.1 respectively. Very clever.

I tried to brush past, but Stan got in the way.

"Sorry, honey. This area is for models only." He pointed at a sign taped to the wall. Bitches!

I tried to brush him away, but he had 4 inches and 40 pounds on me. "Fuck off, Stan. I've got to get ready."

"Ready for what?" sneered Paul.

"Maybe he hasn't heard," said Matthew, relishing every moment. He *almost* had the Versace shoot before I showed up.

"You're out of the show," said Stan.

You'd think that couldn't surprise me, but it did. Reckless, self-destructive behavior was not only tolerated in the modeling world but encouraged. And penalties were practically non-existent. Getting kicked out of a show? I really pissed somebody off this time.

Well, my plan was working.

In hindsight, it's easy to see how much I hated the industry and how much I wanted to get out. The booze and the drugs were just too alluring for me to walk away by myself, so I had to take a wrecking ball to myself and my career.

I caught a train to Vienna. I needed a quiet city to dry out in. This wasn't my first time trying to get sober. I tried AA back in '94, but it was too rigid for my tastes and didn't stick. I tried other things too, but sobriety didn't stick in '94. Or '96. Or '98. I yo-yoed my way through life for almost six years, swinging from the high-highs of party life to the low-lows of detox.

How had I gotten here? Unfortunately, I had thought modeling was "easy money." For a kid who grew up on the street, money was a high priority, so I stuck with the dysfunction and psychosexual deviancy for much longer than I should have. I hated it to my very core, so I numbed myself with sex, drugs, and alcohol. And I had success. And I had some fun. And I convinced myself that everything was okay and that life was good.

But it wasn't. Far from it. I had no dream. No vision. What kind of legacy would I leave behind? Even in Vienna, I managed to get out of hand. One night, I ran into these professional wrestlers in the Blaue Bar at Hotel Sacher.

"That shit's fake!" I exclaimed, looking up at this 6'5" mountain of a man. "I'll prove it. Let me punch you in the chest."

He agreed. What I didn't hear him say was, "As long as I get to hit you back."

I hurt my wrist. He popped a couple of my teeth out.

If I died right then and everyone gathered for my funeral, what would my mom say about me?

"He was a beautiful fuckup," she'd say, wiping her eyes, "but I loved him anyway."

New Year's Eve 1998

After Milan, I moved back to Los Angeles and decided to pursue an acting career. I got a little place in Santa Monica and started taking acting classes. I loved the city and made a bunch of cool new friends.

But I was frustrated too.

It was New Year's Eve, and like most aspiring actors in Hollywood, I was waiting tables. But what really frustrated me was the booze. I'd tried to kick it. I really had. I had been going to AA meetings religiously all year, but it wasn't working for me.

Case and point: I didn't have a girlfriend. Not anymore. Not after last night. Nine months of sobriety down the tubes in a hot mess of vodka-filled rage.

I recognized how destructive alcohol was in my life: it made me an emotional wreck and strained or ruined my personal and professional relationships. If I was going to make it as an actor, I couldn't do it as a drunk.

There was something about AA that stuck. Step Eleven, of the twelve step process, encourages prayer and meditation, which means a lot of different things to a lot of different people, as AA doesn't promote Christianity over other religions, or really promote any religion at all. Some of the guys I saw make good progress were not religious at all, but they were finding comfort and peace through meditation. It was this, that really intrigued me. Something about meditation really drew me in.

I picked up some books and found a little Buddhist community center that offered free classes. I really didn't know what I was doing, but those hours of stillness helped me in a way that the caffeine-driven, nicotine-saturated "Sharing Sessions" at AA never could.

I was waiting for table 12's surf-and-turf to come up when Prince's "1999" came on the radio for about the hundredth time that day.

I was dreamin' when I wrote this, forgive me if it goes astray
But when I woke up this mornin', could've sworn it was
judgment day.

I realized by the time I got out of there, it really would be 1999, and that depressed me deeply. Something had to change.

"Hey, Troy. Happy New Year!"

Julio was a waiter at the restaurant, too. Like me, he was an aspiring actor, and like me, he also struggled with alcohol.

"Check this out," he said, handing me a big manila envelope. "What is it?" I asked.

"It's that meditation course I was telling you about," he smiled. "I am telling you, it's the granddaddy of them all."

Last time we worked together, I mentioned that I was interested in learning more about meditation, and he told me about his life-changing experience: He sat ten days in silence, meditating and "ridding his mind of defilement." After that, he swore he hadn't had a drop to drink. That was two years ago.

On my break, I took the packet out to my car and read about the course. As I looked through the material, I had tears in my eyes. I knew this was something I had to do. Four months later, I sat for ten days of Vipassana meditation.

As I would learn later, there are two types of meditation in Buddhism: Samatha and Vipassana. Samatha promotes concentration and tranquility: you focus on one thing and prevent your mind from wandering. Vipassana focuses on insight: it teaches you to live in the moment, to be aware and to be mindful, it helps you break down illusions and see the world as it really is.

Vipassana is the oldest meditation practice, often attributed to the Buddha himself. It is a gradual – but extremely thorough – process that takes years and years to perfect.

Vipassana examines different aspects of one's existence. It is an ancient, rigorous system with a codified set of exercises that help train your mind to be more aware. More open. More present.

Eventually, I would relearn how to experience the world. How to smell deeply, how to touch fully, how to listen intently. But first I needed to learn to breathe.

The breath work was startling. Something as seemingly simple as breathing is so full of mystery and potential. The riotous ocean that had been my life calmed.

Storm clouds dissipated. Fog lifted. More and more still, breath by breath, day after day, until the sea was as smooth as glass. Tranquility. Bliss. Rapture.

It is impossible to put the experience into words. The only way to understand is to experience it for yourself. Focused breath work has changed my life completely, and I cannot recommend it enough.

The ultimate goal of Vipassana meditation – of Buddhism itself – is liberation. To be free of the shackles of illusion and to experience life as it really is.

But what does that even mean? Shackles of illusions? I've got to admit, I had a healthy dose of skepticism going in. I thought I already saw the world pretty clearly. Sure, I was a fucked-up mess, but I *knew* I was a fucked-up mess.

Everything we experience is the result of how our brain processes the data it receives. Sight, sound, smell, touch – all involve a complex series of chemical reactions in our nervous system, which are translated and given meaning by our brains.

There are more than 100 billion neurons in our nervous system. The body sends way more signals than the brain can reasonably process all at once, so our brains adapt. Over a lifetime we build a huge database of experiences, which our brain stores and cross-references. The first time we do something, it may take a lot of conscious effort. But the more we do it, the more automatic – or subconscious – it becomes. Our brains can scan the data, pull up past experiences, and fill in the rest.

This can be tremendously helpful, allowing us to focus our attention on the important things while the mundane tasks are handled subconsciously. But it can also blind us to the world, especially if we don't know which things in life are important and which are mundane.

Meditation did what AA never could for me. It helped me sober up, sure. But more than that, the mental training I received has helped me experience the world in a whole new way. This journey of self-discovery – of self love – has helped me mentally, physically, emotionally, and spiritually.

As my head began to clear, I started to see the interconnectedness of things. I thought about my time in Milan and I examined my experiences there with more than just insight—I saw those years as a prelude to the journey I was on now. I began to see more clearly how the things I put in my body affected me. I stopped putting drugs and alcohol into my system. I quit smoking. I paid attention to the foods I ate. I also started taking herbs and supplements from Amazon Herb Co. They had a power in them that upgraded my energy field. I could feel them in my loins. They made me horny. Gave me a boner.

I got to know the owner of Amazon Herb Co. pretty well. Amazon John Easterling is a fascinating character. He's a real-life Indiana Jones. Back in the seventies, he went to the Amazon looking for El Dorado – the lost city of gold. The search almost killed him. He was at death's door when some indigenous people took him in and healed him. Since then, John has spent his life studying the biodiversity of the rainforest and learning the secrets of plant medicine. He's become a major figure in the fight to preserve this precious ecosystem. Oh yeah, he's also married to Olivia Newton-John. He found treasure in the Amazon – and it was much more precious than gold.

During that time of my life, I was reading a lot about ancient cultures around the world and their use of psychedelic plant medicine to peel back the veils in their minds and reveal universal truths. In particular, I'd read about Amazonian people using ayahuasca for healing. When I told Amazon John I was interested in experiencing ayahuasca firsthand, he pointed me in the direction of Scott Petersen. Like Amazon John, Scott had a life-altering experience in the Amazon. Now he was living among the Shipibo Indians and healing with ayahuasca.

In 2006, I found myself standing on the curb at the airport in

Pucallpa, Peru, waiting for Scott Petersen – "The Gringo Shaman" – to pick me up.

Scott wasn't at all what I expected.

He rolled up on this motorized rickshaw-looking bike and told me to hop in. As we weaved in and out of traffic, dodging cars and bikes and kids and chickens, he puffed his mapacha cigar and regaled me with stories about everything from the locals to riding broncos in the rodeo.

This guy was more cowboy than holy man, but he was funny as shit.

"Last week," he said, "this 15-foot anaconda came into ceremony and wrapped itself around a shaman."

He took another drag on his cigar and smiled at me as a cloud of *nicotiana rustica* tobacco smoke trailed off behind our rickshaw. "You know what we call that?"

"Shit. Snakes in ceremony?" "That's an Amazon hug."

He laughed a big belly laugh as we pulled up to the banks of the Ucayali River.

"This is as far as the road will take us. We go upriver from here." I climbed out of the rickshaw; feeling jostled and a little green from the mix of gasoline, exhaust fumes, and cigar smoke.

"Don't worry," he winked. "I haven't lost one in ceremony yet." He laughed another one of his belly laughs, frightening a flock of yellow-and-black birds out of the bush and over the mud-brown river.

Going upriver was a journey I'll never forget. Oxygen – literally right from nature's tap – flooded my system. My whole body was viscerally flipped on. Senses on overload. Green had never looked so lush and vibrant before. The smell of flowers I couldn't name seduced my olfactory bulb. My skin glistened and shivered with excitement, and saliva stampeded across my tongue, preparing for some unseen feast. Beaks drummed on trunks, setting down a rhythm to an anthem of life composed and performed in real time by millions of life forces crowding in around the boat.

"That's a caiman," Scott said, pointing at a three-foot long alligator-like reptile slipping into the water for a fish dinner. "Mostly docile but be careful not to step on one. They can be nasty little buggers."

I wouldn't say I was in a state of fear, but my sympathetic nervous system was on high alert. Fight or flight had kicked into high gear. I was not at the top of the food chain, and there were any number of things (seen and unseen) that might like to slice me open and eat me. Or worse...colonize my intestines and devour me from the inside out.

Scott looked at the sky and announced, "I think we'll do ceremony tonight. How much do you know about the medicine?"

Medicine? Who the fuck was he kidding? Ayahuasca was a drug, a hallucinogen with a reputation that set it aside from other psychedelics. I've got to admit, I had more than a little trepidation about this.

Four days earlier, I had been up near Machu Picchu doing a San Pedro ceremony. I prayed to the four directions and drank the sacrament of that trippy cactus. I didn't go "deep," but it was definitely powerful enough to peel back my consciousness.

The next day, I confided in the shaman.

"Look," I said. "I haven't been drinking for many years. I don't use drugs or anything like that. I am about to go to the Amazon and drink ayahuasca, but I have some trepidation."

He nodded and reflected for a moment. Then he said, "Your trepidation is normal. Ayahuasca is not child's play."

Scott had this preternatural ability to read people. It was like my thoughts were written in a bubble over my head.

"Ah," he said, taking a long drag on his cigar. "You don't think ayahuasca is medicine." I shrugged my shoulders. And thus began my education.

"Ayahuasca is the mother of all healing plants in the Amazon," he said. "The beautiful thing about ayahuasca is that it heals us on multiple levels. It heals the body, cleanses the blood, the liver, and the gallbladder. It clears the emotional field by allowing us to process our old traumas and liberate ourselves from these things. And it also brings our energy into the third eye and the crown chakra, allowing us to experience the celestial realm."

I could tell he loved and admired this plant from the way he spoke about it. There was the kind of reverence in his words that you only hear when someone is talking about a great person.

"It also has an opening effect for the other medicinal plants, and when you take ayahuasca, you'll be more receptive to the other plants. That's why, when we're healing someone with chronic disease, we'll first give them ayahuasca, even if it's at a very small dosage, so we can have that spirit present. That will open doors for the other plants to come in and have a more vital impact on whatever we're working on. It also opens up people's spirits so that they're willing to accept healing because many people have a vested interest in being sick or weak."

What the hell did he mean by that?

Scott seemed to read my thoughts again, like I was the Sunday comics.

"There's nothing more frightening than being completely well, because then you have to take responsibility for the world around you."

Growing up on the streets and experiencing everything I had as a model had conditioned me to approach everything – and everyone – with a healthy dose of skepticism. I can smell BS a mile away, and sometimes in the big city, it's the only thing you *can* smell.

I *knew* that Scott was authentic. He truly believed what he was telling me. It came from a place of honesty and goodwill. He wasn't trying to sell me. He was trying to teach me.

But with ayahuasca, words are just shadows and mist. There is no knowing without experiencing. That's why I had made this journey to begin with. Over the past six years, I'd cleaned up my body, my mind, and my spirit. I was learning to love myself and soaking up all the information I could about health, nutrition, and fitness.

I was beginning the journey that would lead me to be *RippedAt50*.

What dream and purpose did I have for my own life? What legacy would I leave behind? Meditation was miraculous. It brought calmness and clarity, and my life was coming into focus. But many cultures throughout history had also used psychedelics to strip away the ego and see the universe as it really is. Using psychedelics for clarity may sound counterintuitive, but meditation had taught me to keep an open mind.

And then I heard about ayahuasca. Psychedelics aren't my thing, but I was fascinated by the stories I'd read. Was it really possible that some tiny molecule in my brain could open up a door to a different consciousness? To help me to escape from the walls I'd built up in my mind and perceive the world through a different lens?

I was intrigued.

"Make sure you go with intention," my hippie friends told me. And so I did. My intention in going to the Amazon was to connect with the divine feminine in all its facets and to open up my heart. Empathy, intuition, community, and collaboration were all aspects I could improve on.

But could ayahuasca really help bring my legacy into focus? Could it show me who I really was, and where I was going?

When we arrived at the center, Scott took me on a tour.

"The Shipibo have a legend about ayahuasca," he said, showing me the plant climbing up a bamboo trellis. "Long ago, the tribe was dependent on a very old shaman for all their healing. The people came to him and said, 'What are we going to do when you die? Who will heal us?' And the shaman (who was about 120 years old) said, 'I am going to die very soon, but don't worry. When I die, don't bury me in the ground. Take my body and tie it to a tree branch, and out of my body will grow a vine that will teach you to be your own prophet, priest, and healer too.'"

Scott stepped across the path and gently touched another plant. "And when my wife dies, take her body and bury it at the base of the tree, and from her body will grow the complimentary plant – the *chacruna* plant."

"And if you cook our two bodies together," Scott smiled, pointing to a pot simmering on a nearby fire, "you will come up with a brew that will make you a healer."

It had been a long day, and Scott could see the weariness in my shoulders.

"You should get some rest. It's going to be a big night." He showed me to my bungalow, then disappeared to prepare for the ceremony.

I meditated for a while as the lullaby of the forest called me to slumber. The words of the San Pedro ceremony shaman floated through my consciousness: Ayahuasca is not child's play.

I woke feeling refreshed and more alive than I can ever remember feeling. Excited, yet relaxed. Calm, but with butterflies in my stomach. The perfect balance of different energies.

A little after 7 PM, an elderly Shipibo woman informed me it was time. She led me to the ceremony house as the color faded from the sky and the first stars began to appear.

Scott opened up the ceremony by praying in the four directions, and then administered the medicine. It was bitter and *really* thick. The taste made me gag, but I managed to get it down.

"I've heard that ayahuasca can make you shit and puke," I told Scott as I waited for the medicine to kick in.

"Yeah," he smiled. "That's true. It does have strong purgative powers."

At Scott's direction, another shaman began whistling, then singing in a low guttural voice.

"Shaman sing the icarus – the magic songs – to push your energy up into your crown chakra and help prepare you for healing and awareness." He shook a chakapa, a sort of rattle made from a dried-out bush. "But I am not much of a singer," he confessed blowing mapacho smoke over me, "so you are blessed to have him sing the icaro."

The jungle joined in the icaro, fluting, and cawing, and beating out a rhythm that I could feel in my gut. Sacred geometry fractured into swirling kaleidoscopes as insects started to buzz in my ear.

A lot of people talk about seeing God as being filled with the divine spirit and communing with angels. Not me. Forty-five minutes into this thing, I was in the bathroom shitting myself silly and fighting the urge to puke.

I've done about thirty ayahuasca ceremonies since that first one. There are always some hallucinations, but they're always at the periphery of my consciousness. For me, it always comes down to my gut. There I am, alone with my intestines, feeling the medicine work its way into my core.

"It's good," Scott said, blowing rose water over me as the icaro moved into higher octaves. "Sometimes you have to go through hell to heal."

Ain't that the truth!

Hour after hour, the medicine worked its way through me as the icaro climbed and climbed, pushing my energy higher and higher. Kaleidoscopic eyeballs peered down at me, ugly and angry, as the bad bacteria in my gut writhed and squirmed. An unstoppable tsunami of ayahuasca was flushing them away.

The memories and feelings I'd carried for so long started to pass through me. Anger at being beaten by my stepfather. Alone on the streets. Hungry and stinking. Modeling in Milan. Paris. New York. Psychosexual manipulation and betrayal. Drinking. Drugs.

Numbness. Escape. No...not escape. Denial.

Icaro rises higher. Birds' sensual songs. Sacred geometry. DNA. Drumming. Anger. Rejection. Champagne. Cocaine. Hip hop. Hippocrates.

All disease starts in the gut.

Stress. Worry. Anxiety. Fear. Always in the gut. My bowels were writhing. Icaro higher and higher. And then clarity. Knowing.

Have you ever known something without a shadow of a doubt? 100% sure? Without question? Absolute?

I felt it. I knew it. And I started laughing.

"Welcome to paradise," said Scott , smiling down at me.

I *knew* it. Which means I always knew it, but just somehow forgot.

How could I forget something so integral? It was like forgetting my own name. I laughed until my sides hurt.

Scott laughed too, his big belly laugh. And the birds joined in. Harsh and liquid sounds. Caws and screeches.

It was a cosmic joke. And there, on the celestial plane, everyone was in on it. I am Troy Casey, the Certified Health Nut.

As I floated above the canopy of the forest, I could see below me a temple in a clearing. The structure was ancient and beautiful beyond anything I had ever seen. As I circled lower and lower, I counted nine pillars holding aloft a massive stone structure. As I got closer, I could see the intricately carved faces of everyone I knew.

I could see one of the pillars leaning badly, causing the domed structure on top to tilt precariously to the west, but fortunately the remaining pillars bore the weight and kept the temple from collapsing.

Ayahuasca works in me through "knowing." I can't explain how I know what I know, but my experiences with the medicine have filled me with knowledge. In that moment, I knew the temple was me. I knew the pillars were the essential aspects that supported my life. And I knew that if I ignored the pillars, my life would collapse.

I alighted on the ground and walked barefoot through the temple, I stopped to look at each pillar.

The first pillar bore the image of a sleeping babe at the base. It seemed impossibly narrow at the bottom, incapable of holding the massive boulders that loomed above. But as the pillar rose from the infant, it sprang into wondrous shapes that grew organically around the central column, reaching to the ceiling in beautiful lines that were indescribably intricate. I knew that this pillar represented my legacy. The pillar imbued the entire temple with its DNA, and each of the other pillars seemed to be built to support this one. Why am I here? What is my purpose in life? What legacy will I leave behind?

The second pillar was not stone, but a tree trunk that radiated with life. From the tree, all manner of fruits and vegetables grew, gleaming with vitality. I sat and ate the food that the tree provided, and I was nourished.

The next pillar I came to seemed to be made of mist, and I lay down to sleep deeply beside it. I dreamed of a baby girl named Athena, and my heart was filled with a love that made me want to weep with joy.

I awoke feeling strong, looking at the fourth pillar floating above me in the clouds. I reached for a vine and began climbing. I walked for many miles, and then swam across a clear blue lake to finally stand in its shadow. The movement of my limbs felt strong and righteous.

Not far from there was the fifth pillar. I sat and breathed deeply under a canopy of leaves that sprang from its living structure, and my mind was clear and bright.

Next, I sat with my back to the sixth pillar and looked out on the panorama before me. The air was crystal clear, and I could see for miles and miles. When I focused my thoughts to the east and imagined a cathedral there, one sprang up in the distance. When I looked to the west and wondered how the people would cross the wide river, a bridge stretched from one shore to the next. Everything my mind conceived blossomed into existence.

Later, I found myself climbing a spiral staircase that encircled the seventh pillar. This column was made up of people I knew. Each person in his or her own way was holding up some part of the dome overhead. Some areas were so dark, I could barely see who was underneath, while others shone so brightly, I could not look at them.

The next pillar stood at the mouth of a spring, its water cascading down, feeding the temple. Water, I knew, was the source of life, and this temple would perish without it. I drank deeply there and was refreshed and invigorated.

Finally, I came to the last pillar, which sprang out of the earth itself. Vines from this pillar crawled and stretched and climbed across the floor and ceiling, becoming entwined with each of the other columns. A life force flowed from nature itself into the temple.

This is the vision – the knowing – that ayahuasca gave me in the Amazonian jungle in 2006. But like waking from a vivid dream, the details became jumbled in my waking mind and drifted into my subconscious, just out of my reach. It took me several years to unpack all that I saw and everything I learned.

In the coming chapters, I am going to lay out – as best as I can – what I know. I've organized this book into the 9 Pillars, which are:

1. The Legacy Pillar
2. The Food Pillar
3. The Rest Pillar
4. The Movement Pillar
5. The Breath Pillar
6. The Thought Pillar
7. The Relationship Pillar
8. The Water Pillar
9. The Nature Pillar

In each chapter, I'll share my personal story, then describe some of the steps you can take to build and strengthen your own pillars.

RippedAt50 is not a diet book. It's not an exercise book, either. It's a book about living optimally. Yeah, I have six-pack abs and you can, too, if you really want them. But that's not the legacy I want to leave behind.

I believe that health is the birthright of all people. Sadly, recent studies have shown than more than 95% of humans on this planet are living with some form of illness. Dig deeper, and you'll see that the vast majority of disease and illness can be tied directly to the choices we make. Smoking, alcohol, and drug use/abuse are major contributors. But so are diet and exercise choices. As we will discuss in The Rest Pillar chapter, humans are the only animal species that willingly deprive themselves of sleep, and the impact can be dire. Add to that the wholesale changes in agriculture, the explosion of GMOs and glyphosate in our food, the contamination of our air, water, and soil, the pervasive negative impact of media and social media on our emotional wellbeing, and our disconnection with nature, and it's no surprise to see that we're suffering from the choices we've made.

Unlike my ayahuasca-fueled vision of the Temple of Troy, the jungle I actually live in is made of concrete. Over the past 13 years, I've read thousands of books on health. I've studied under some of the smartest and most knowledgeable people on the planet. I've ventured to remote corners of the world to learn secrets I couldn't read about. Now, I teach the workshops, write the books, and work with my clients to help them understand their health better.

On the one hand, there is a lot of science involved and – full disclosure – I am not a scientist. But I've applied the scientific method to my life. Through careful observation, I've developed hypotheses, conducted experiments, and measured the results. I have learned through life experience that my own cognitive assumptions can distort how I interpret my observations, and I keep a healthy skepticism about my own observations. Decades of meditation have helped me see the world as it is, not as I would like it to be.

I've refined or eliminated hypotheses as the outcomes of my life play out for all to see. I am my own petri dish. But I am *RippedAt50*. My stomach is flat, and my brain is intact. I've never felt better in my life.

What I've learned has helped me, and I hope it can help you too.

Legacy is about having a dream and purpose for your life and leaving behind something of value. While each of the 9 Pillars is important, legacy is arguably the most vital.

Without dream and purpose, all the other pillars are diminished. Building your Legacy Pillar starts with a mission/vision statement. While this statement should ideally only be a few sentences, it may take you years to develop and perfect. Here's how to start:

"I am" Statements

In my workshops or when working one-on-one with my clients, I use a couple of exercises that help them begin to articulate their legacy. First, I start with "I am" statements. These aspirational statements aim to expose who you really want to be. To start, complete this "simple" statement:

I am _____.

Consider the following questions:

What do you want to do? Who do you want to be?

Write down as many as you can, then start to see the connections between them.

Do you see a theme or pattern developing? Can you pick the one statement that most closely identifies who you want to be?

Mission/Vision Exercises

These exercises help you think about what is most important to you and begin to understand what legacy you want to leave behind. Start by answering these questions.

- If you won the lottery right now, and money was no object, what would you do with your life?
- If you died, and everyone was gathered for your funeral, what would your mother, father, husband, wife, brother, sister, best friend, etc., say about you?

If those two exercises don't produce useful results, try a different angle. Instead of hope and aspirations, let's look at your fears. Are you afraid of being poor? Or of being alone? Complete the following statements:

- I am NOT _____.
- I don't want to _____.
- My biggest fear is _____.

Now let's use the completed statements to help us answer the mission/vision questions. If you don't want to be lonely, what can you do to prevent it?

Personal Mission/Vision Statement

All of this work leads to your personal mission/vision statement. The statement should be short and concise. You should be able to commit it to memory and recite it. If you're finding that your statement isn't coming so easily, don't be discouraged. I didn't develop mine overnight – it has been a long and ever-evolving process. Here is my personal mission/vision statement:

I am a humble, kind, and gentle man. My mission is to raise human consciousness and change all systems. My vision is clean air, water, soil, and equitable systems for all mankind...in my lifetime.

FOOD

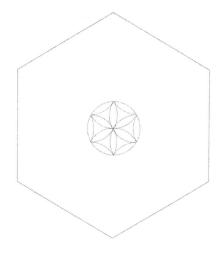

CHAPTER TWO

"Let food be thy medicine and medicine be thy food."

Hippocrates

Summer of 1989

MY MODELING CAREER was taking off. I left California and found myself in Milan working in this strange, exciting new industry. Models were celebrities in Milan. I am not saying I was a celebrity myself, but I had joined an elite group of mortals and demigods in this Neo-Roman myth-building culture.

I was a scrapper from the street with a high school education and three years of community college. But I had a look that got reactions, and I was a pretty good bullshitter, which made up for my lack of polish.

I didn't speak Italian, but I didn't really need to. Almost everybody spoke English anyway, so I picked up the basics and faked the rest.

In hindsight, modeling was a really hard way to make a living. It's not like a real job. You book a shoot and get paid what seems like a lot of money, but then you have to scramble and hustle and sweet talk (or worse) your way to the next gig before the money runs out. But when you're surrounded by a bunch of people who live the same reality, it really doesn't seem strange at all. You get comfortable in your bubble. Happy even. And for someone who grew up dumpster diving just to eat, this was a huge step up.

On the street, I had to worry about food, shelter, and safety. In Milan, none of those things was a concern. I was living in a hotel with a bunch of other models and had no trouble covering my living expenses. Safety wasn't a concern. Models in Milan were surrounded by several layers of protection, which was something I had never experienced before.

First, there was a general cultural attitude. Models in Milan are like actors in Hollywood. You gain a certain social status by appearing in glossy magazine ads, billboards, and bus sides. Anyone would KILL to take your place.

If you score a magazine cover or – even better – a national TV campaign, you are a star. You become a household name. Everyone loves you. The world is your oyster. Like a Botticelli painting, you stand half-naked for the entire world to see, as the gods of fashion blow your hair for dramatic effect and cloak you in the finest of garments. You are a thing to be respected. Revered. Worshipped.

Then there was the mob. Models are currency in Milan, and the mob doesn't miss a trick. Every club owner wanted models at the bar and on the dance floor. It was a big attraction. Everybody wanted to party with the beautiful people. So the mob facilitated what we used to call "Dancing for Dollars" parties.

No one messed with us at the clubs. It was bad for business, and that wasn't tolerated.

The main duty for the "runners" (as I called the mob guys who facilitated these things) was to keep drunk and/or horny guys off the women. But the male models were part of the package and under their protection too.

They didn't act as personal bodyguards, mind you. I learned the hard way that if you got too drunk and crossed the line, they'd stand around laughing as you got your ass kicked in the parking lot.

The first week I was in Milan, I fell in with a couple of guys from Australia who took me to one of these Dancing for Dollars parties. Only I thought we were just going to a bar.

Chris and Jack had been doing pretty well in their new modeling careers – their muscular good looks and easy-going Aussie charm had made them darlings of the fashion scene.

"You should come with, Troy," said Chris. "We'll introduce you to Krystal."

"She's producing," cut in Jack. "She's an old friend from Brisbane. Good gal to know." "Yeah, sure. Thanks, guys. That would be great!"

I needed friends like these. "Can I buy you a drink?" I asked, naively. They both laughed.

"Come on, rookie," Chris joked, jabbing me in the ribs with his elbow. "Models don't pay for drinks around here."

"Food either," said Jack, pointing to a door marked *Private*.

"Free pizza and snacks in there." He got the barmaid's attention and she brought us three beers.

"This is 'Dancing for Dollars,'" said Jack, gesturing around the room.

"We come in the back door, drink for free, and enjoy all that the underbelly of Milan has to offer," laughed Chris. "All we have to do is shake our asses on the dance floor a little."

They shook their muscular Aussie asses all night and drank like fish, and I joined in with abandon.

6:00 am rolled around, but they were looking fresh and rested, ready to conquer the day. What is it about Australians?

We rolled into the studio at 6:45 am and the place was already buzzing. Like the club the night before, these guys seemed to know everyone, and everyone seemed to love them. They introduced me around. Here I was, the new kid at school, and I'd already fallen in with two of the popular kids! I couldn't help but have a little strut in my step. I was going to love it here.

"Oy, Krystal," yelled Jack, whistling above the din. She smiled and crossed to meet us. "Oy, fuckers," she said, kissing them both.

"Krystal, we want you to meet Troy," said Chris. "We heard you were looking for a fresh face, and he just got here from California."

Krystal looked me up and down sharply. The smile faded from her face.

"Honey, you're too fat," she said, and then scooted off to talk to the photographer. Jack and Chris chuckled and smacked me on the back.

"No worries, mate," Chris said. "I think she likes you."

"Me too," laughed Jack. "Otherwise she would have said..." "No good," they both said in unison.

"'No good' means no way ever," said Jack.

"'Too fat' means you've got a chance," said Chris encouragingly. "You just need to lose a few pounds."

"Maybe too much pizza last night," Chris laughed, patting my belly.

"We'll see you tonight, right?" asked Jack as they made their way to the dressing rooms.

"Sure," I replied, trying to keep a smile on my face. "See you tonight."

They disappeared into the crowd, and I stood there in the midst of the hustle and bustle with the words ringing in my ears. *Honey, you're too fat.*

I was no Botticelli painting. I was more Edvard Munch, holding my skeletal head between my ghostly hands, eyes popping, mouth stretched in an eternal scream, filled with anxiety and self-doubt.

Fat? What the hell! I needed to lose weight, but how? I'd never had to diet before. I'd seen how a lot of models do it: starve themselves to death. But I had seen the impact of those diets on others. I had to take a different route. Whatever was happening inside of my body was affecting the way I looked—my face showed signs of my poor digestion and inflammation. I needed to get healthy if only to look healthy. I walked around the city for hours, sweating and thinking. Eventually, I found myself in an American bookstore, buying everything I could find on nutrition.

Like the average American kid growing up in the seventies and eighties, I was educated on nutrition through the food pyramid. I thought that Cap'n Crunch and Pop-Tarts were a healthy part of a balanced breakfast, and TV dinners were the perfect solution for a busy lifestyle. But in Italy, people didn't eat like that. They went to local farmers markets and bought real food, and on average they were thirty pounds lighter than their American counterparts. I started to give up the processed foods in favor of fresh fruits and vegetables. I learned the nutritional value of above-ground vegetables and grass-fed ruminants.

As a model who was drinking a lot, I paid more attention to water weight too. I learned that dandelion was not only a diuretic, it was also good for my liver. I started to amass a toolkit of herbs and supplements that helped me stay trim and provided the vitamins, minerals, and nutrients my body needed. I learned about juicing, fasting, and cleansing too. After my first ten-day cleanse, I looked in the mirror, and I looked younger and trimmer than I had in years. I was hooked!

Over the 30 years that have passed since that rude awakening of being called fat, I've continued to educate myself and perfect my diet and nutrition. The science is deep and vast, and I could write a whole book on the subject, but for our purposes here, I am going to boil my knowledge into the essential information you need to get started.

The Science of Your Gut

If you think you know everything about nutrition because you took some biology classes in school and learned about the food pyramid, it's time to go back to school. We have traveled light-years since then.

You may have heard of the Human Genome Project. This $30B research project, funded by the U.S. Government, began in 1990. The goal was to map all the genes in the human genome, and the work was completed in 2003. What we learned from this project has propelled our understanding of how the body works at a cellular level.

Four years after the human genome research was completed, the National Institute of Health (NIH) launched the Human Microbiome Project, which set out to map the microbes that live in the human body.

Before the study, little was known about the microbes that live inside us. We didn't know how many different kinds of microbes there were. We didn't have names for them, and we certainly didn't know what impact they had on our health.

Everything has changed.

Scientists estimate there are more than 10,000 species of microbes living in (and on) humans! They also learned that the colonizing microbes contribute more genes that are responsible for human survival than human genes. In fact, scientists estimate that bacterial protein-coding genes are 360 times more abundant than human genes!

Your microbiome – the community of microbes that lives in you – plays a bigger role in your health than your human genes do. This is not just one doctor or scientist coming to this conclusion. Hundreds of research teams from all around the world have published peer-reviewed articles on this exciting new science.

Nutrition at a Cellular Level

It's an interesting paradox that humans are made up of about 10% human cells and 90% bacterial cells (we can argue the actual percentages, but the fact remains that bacteria cells far outnumber human cells in our body).

As a rule of thumb, about 85% of the 10,000 or so species in our guts should be "good" bacteria, and 15% should be "bad" bacteria.

Hold on – why do you want 15% bad bacteria?

Simply put, your immune system needs bad bacteria to help you survive. By encountering – and learning to deal with – these bad bacteria in small doses, your body prepares itself to fight off disease. The world can be a dangerous place, and your body has ingenious ways of defending itself.

"Dysbiosis" is the scientific term for a microbial imbalance and, in the context of this book, it refers to the imbalance of "good" and "bad" bacteria in our guts. Commercial food, which is sprayed with herbicides and pesticides and is full of chemical additives, can feed the bad bacteria while starving the good bacteria. This, in turn, affects the release of hormones and receptor sites throughout your body.

The "Gut Brain"

Have you ever had a "gut instinct?" Something within you, at your very core, that "tells" you something? You don't know how you know, but you KNOW! It turns out that this saying has a basis in science.

The vagus nerve connects your brain and your gut. Extending through your neck, chest, and abdomen, it helps control mood, immune response, digestion, and heart rate.

This connection between your brain and your gut is known as the gut-brain axis. It provides two-way communication between your brain and your gut. The most important job of the vagus nerve is to send information about the gut, liver, heart, and lungs to the brain.

When it comes to food intake, the vagus nerve is responsible for sending all kinds of information from the gut to the brain, including feelings of hunger and satiety ("satiety" means feeling sated or satisfied; in other words, NOT feeling hungry). This means that your cravings for food are driven not by your brain, but by your gut. Put another way, the alien microbes in your gut are deciding what you should eat.

Ever hear of the zombie apocalypse? We may be living it already! The gut brains are in charge!!!

I imagine you're as skeptical as I was when I first encountered this concept. How can you call a collection of microbes a "brain," anyway? Let's talk about that.

Your brain is the center of your nervous system. It has about 100 billion neurons that can be "electrically excited" in several ways, including by chemical transmitters. Take, for instance, the chemical serotonin. Serotonin can affect your mood, appetite, sleep, body temperature, and more. It also regulates your intestines and is important for digestion.

Would it surprise you to learn that approximately 90% of the serotonin in your body is produced in your gut? Now think about 10,000+ different kinds of bacteria creating a complex chemical stew in your gut, activating some genes, inhibiting others, sending all sorts of messages to your brain.

The bad bacteria want different molecules than the good ones. Your gut instinct changes. You start to crave carbs. You start to crave sugar. The bad bacteria need them. They *demand* them. Thus begins a downward spiral. Guts become bloated. Inflammation occurs, and with it a host of health issues.

Glyphosate

Glyphosate is a broad-spectrum systemic herbicide and crop desiccant. Monsanto brought it to market in 1974 under the brand name Roundup. Glyphosate inhibits a particular enzyme in plants (5-enolpyruvylshikimate-3-phosphate for those of you going for extra credit). Without this enzyme, the plant's reproductive and immune systems are destroyed, and the plant dies.

Monsanto also engineered crops in a laboratory to make them tolerant to glyphosate. These "Roundup Ready" crops allow farmers to spray their fields freely with glyphosate – killing the weeds but leaving the crops alone.

From 1974 through 2016, the use of glyphosate-based herbicides

(GBHs) has increased 100-fold worldwide; it is the most used herbicide in U.S. agriculture. But don't worry, it's all perfectly safe. You see, the particular shikimate pathway that glyphosate uses to kill plants doesn't exist in humans, so it can't affect you (at least that's what Monsanto would have you believe). But if you're using the scientific method, you should approach that last statement with a healthy dose of skepticism.

Remember the microbiome, and the 10,000+ species of alien microbes that live in your gut and control more gene expression in your body than your human cells do? Well, some of them *do* have shikimate pathways that make them vulnerable to glyphosate.

What does that mean exactly?

Well, the truth is, we're still trying to find out. We're living this planetary experiment right now. There are hundreds of studies out there linking glyphosate to negative health effects.

I believe we've fundamentally changed the food that goes into our bodies, and it is having a catastrophic effect. GMOs, pesticides and herbicides, highly processed foods full of chemicals – these things are literally killing us. I could fill another thousand pages with scientific data, but let's cut to the chase.

What is the solution?

#JERF

Just eat real food. That's it. Pretty simple, right?

Well...it takes some practice, but it's not that hard. I've been living it for a couple of decades now, and I feel great.

#JERF means you should be able to recognize food as you hold it in your hand and put it on your plate. It shouldn't come in a box, or a can, or a jar – but if it does, read the ingredients. If you can't pronounce it, don't put it in your mouth!

But not all "real" food is equal either. Here's how I rank them:

1. Wild
2. Biodynamic (Demeter)
3. Farmer Direct
4. Organic
5. USDA

Wild

The best food for our bodies is wild food. Food in the wild is the purest because it is in the ideal ecosystem. If you can hunt or fish your own wild food, that's ideal. Wild is the exact natural design of evolution. It uses the energy from the sun, the minerals from the earth, as well as all the adaptation markers. It uses insects, weather, and other things that make the plant or animal genetically stronger (as opposed to cultivated). Wild food often has more unique photochemistry and is more nutritionally dense.

By contrast, the food industry tries to systematically improve yield through science, often through a very unnatural process. They feed animals grains that they are not supposed to eat, simply to fatten them up and increase profits. They splice the genes of plants in a laboratory to try and gain an unfair advantage over nature.

When plants are in the wild, they must build their own natural pesticides, herbicides, and protection. These are what we find in the alkaloids and terpenes that have medicinal components that help human beings.

"Wild" is in a league of its own with natural selection and natural evolution. It is strong, vital, and adapted to a specific environment. For example, buriti oil comes from a palm that grows along the Amazon River. It not only gets high heat from the equatorial sun but also from sunlight that bounces off the river. The plant species needs to protect itself from that much radiation, so it creates the highest concentrated source of beta carotene, which is a natural antioxidant. When you find that in skin care or in nutrition, those natural elements are available to interface into your biochemistry.

Other examples are venison, elk, or wild boar. These are wild animals that are typically in a natural environment. In our culture, we've chosen to eat domesticated chicken, beef, and pork for years. We have been eating these products without knowing the direct effect on our health.

It is vital to know as much as you can about the quality of the wild food you eat. Choosing wild food, in alignment with the best ecosystem, with natural elements, is ideal. Natural elements in the wild help us adapt.

If you can, forage your own "wild." If that is not an option, you may find a local company that will do it for you.

Biodynamic With Demeter Certification

The next best level of nutrition is biodynamic. There are three dominant organic certifiers out there, each of which has different standards. Demeter was the first to establish an organic certification program in 1928 and is the largest and most recognized standard today (certification is difficult to achieve and must be renewed annually).

Demeter's "biodynamic" certification requires biodiversity and ecosystem preservation, soil husbandry, livestock integration, prohibition of genetically engineered organisms, and viewing the farm as a living "holistic organism."

Biodynamic farming was pioneered by Rudolf Steiner, who also created Waldorf education. Steiner's biodynamic farming works with the energy of the celestial bodies, the minerals and rocks in the soil, planting at certain cycles, crop rotation, fallowing, and composting.

This process and these factors are critical components of biodynamic farming. A lot of the organic certifications only require there to be no spraying or chemical synthetics used on the farm. Biodynamics is the highest form of organics because it's all about maintaining the highest-quality soil and getting the microorganisms at a very high level.

Choosing to improve health and nutrition is about continually trying to source the highest-level and best quality food that you can.

Farmer Direct

The next food quality level is farmer direct. Find local farmers and talk to them directly. They are typically very honest people and will tell you how they grow. If they're not growing with chemical pesticides and herbicides, they should be very open about it. If they don't have the certification, just have a conversation and find out if they are using chemical pesticides and herbicides. You deserve to know what you are putting in your body. You can source your food directly and have a relationship with your farmer and your food.

Organic

The next level is organic. Remember that there are different certifiers with many different criteria. Oregon Tilth and Quality Assurance are some of the highest levels of organics. If you're interested, you can certainly research more about the different standards and educate yourself on what is right for you.

The bottom line is that you are looking for organic foods. And, as you probably know, if the food is organic, it is most likely going to be more expensive than non-organic alternatives. Is it worth the price? To me, there is no question. I've observed firsthand the difference all of these levels of food have on my body. My health is of utmost importance to me, and I will pay a premium not to have my food sprayed with poison.

I have no doubt there are people out there who may be able to survive – even thrive – eating commercial food. I think they are rare, that they are genetic anomalies. I am not one of them. My body has clear, observable, measurable reactions to commercial food and operates at a much higher level on organics.

I find it ironic that "organic" is what my grandparents called "food." Just eat real food!

USDA Organic

The next level is USDA Organic. USDA has a much lower standard than other certifiers, and unfortunately the bar seems to sink further and further each year. USDA used to require seven years without pesticides, commercial fertilizers, and other toxic compounds. Now, however, the period has been shortened to three years, and other safeguards have been eliminated, too.

The problem with commercialized food is that it is sprayed with pesticides and herbicides. We've already talked about glyphosate and the havoc it can wreak. You've probably also heard about colony collapse of bees, which is a startling and potentially devastating new ecological development. But beyond the headline-grabbing impacts, we're seeing countless other flora and fauna being annihilated around farmland. The pesticides and herbicides go into the water. They go into the soil. They go into the air. And they find their way into our bodies with, I believe, devastating consequences.

The Four White Devils

There are four "staples" of the average diet that could be playing havoc with your health. They are so commonplace in the world we live in and the food being offered to us that the danger they pose is real and significant. I call these threats to our health "The Four White Devils." They are:

1. White salt
2. White sugar
3. White flour
4. White pasteurized dairy

Let's take a look at the hell each one of these can play on your health.

White Salt

Common table salt is a processed food. Stripped of all the minerals that are present in natural salt, this white devil is produced in a lab and typically full of chemicals that can be detrimental to your health. Most table salt includes anti-caking agents to keep it from clumping. Some anti-caking agents include aluminum, which can potentially be carcinogenic. Table salt also contains iodine. If you eat fresh food grown in mineral-rich soil, you should get all the iodine necessary for your body and not need to supplement it through this artificial method.

Too much (or too little) sodium in your diet can be harmful. Since salt is the most common source of sodium in your diet, and since processed foods are high in sugar and salt content, you should just eat real food (#JERF) and use Celtic sea salt instead of table salt.

White Sugar

Much has been written about this white devil. Too much sugar in your diet can cause a host of health problems including increased risks of obesity, diabetes, and heart conditions. Sugar can negatively impact your immune system, accelerate aging, promote tooth decay and gum disease, impair cognition, and increase stress. Processed white sugar is typically heavily sprayed with pesticides and can contain glyphosate. Studies show that people who consume the most sugar have the highest deficiencies of essential nutrients – especially vitamins A, C, B-12, and calcium.

Avoid eating processed food and try not to artificially sweeten your food. There are so many delicious foods that are naturally sweet! If you must sweeten your foods, try Stevia instead of sugar. Stevia is a natural sweetener extracted from *Stevia rebaudiana*, which is grown in South America. It contains zero calories and isn't linked to weight gain or any known adverse health effects.

White Flour

If you were an evil scientist looking to create an "anti-food" full of harmful effects, you might just develop processed white flour to do the trick. White flour is processed "food" at its worst. Stripped of all nutritional value and devoid of vitamins and minerals, this white devil packs a powerful, unhealthy punch.

Processed foods (such as bread, pasta, chips, crackers, cereals, cookies, and cakes) are high in processed white flour and are commonly called "junk foods." These nutrient-impoverished foods are commonly paired with the other white devils and rob your body of the nutrition it needs. White flour is also a source of gluten that can lead to more ill health effects.

White Pasteurized Dairy

Despite claims to the contrary from various dairy associations, pasteurized white milk has no scientifically proven health benefits. While your body does need calcium, potassium, protein, and fats that are in cow's milk, most scientists agree you are better off getting them from other sources (such as vegetables, fruits, beans, whole grains, nuts, and seeds).

In fact, this white devil may be the source of health issues including allergies, sinus problems, and constipation. Evolution didn't engineer us to digest the milk of cows, and for many of us the negative impacts far outweigh any potential benefits. And even those of us who can tolerate cow's milk may benefit from removing it from our diets. My advice is to try removing dairy from your diet for a couple of weeks and see how you feel. If you notice improvements in your sinuses, headaches, bowel movements, energy, and/or weight, maybe dairy isn't right for you (I seldom have dairy, but when I do, I use unpasteurized dairy from Jersey cows).

The food choices you make every day affect how you live your life. Not just whether you are fat or thin, but *every* aspect of your life. Food can affect your mood and thoughts, impact your relationship with yourself, with others, and with the world you live in. I have found a direct correlation between food and happiness.

Building Your Food Pillar

"You are what you eat." No truer words were ever spoken. The fuel you put into your body has a profound impact on your health and longevity. Here are a few tips to help you build your Nutrition Pillar:

Stop Paying to Poison Yourself

Avoid pesticides and herbicide-laden foods, and steer clear of fake sugar, fake fats, and coloring and preservatives.

Just Eat Real Food (#JERF)

You should be able to recognize food as you hold it in your hand and put it on your plate. It shouldn't come in a box, or a can, or a jar – but if it does, read the ingredients. If you can't pronounce it, don't put it in your mouth!

But not all real food is equal either. Here's how I rank them:

1. Wild
2. Biodynamic (Demeter)
3. Farmer Direct
4. Organic
5. USDA

Try to get the highest-quality food you can. I know it is more expensive, but hey, you're worth it. Focus on **above-ground vegetables** (such as lettuce, spinach, green beans, broccoli, and peppers) and **grass-fed ruminants** (such as cattle, goats, sheep, and deer).

Avoid the **Four White Devils:**

1. White salt
2. White sugar
3. White flour
4. White pasteurized dairy

These are all inflammatory agents and can disrupt your digestion, immune system, stress levels, hormones, and sleep. In a perfect world, you might do away almost completely with sugar, flour, and dairy and use salt sparingly. If you include any of these things in your diet, try these instead:

- Celtic sea salt
- Stevia
- Alternative flours from nuts or seeds, or gluten-free whole grains
- Non-pasteurized dairy from Jersey cows

Also, avoid corn and soy, which are also inflammatory agents. Nuts, grains, and legumes contain phytic acid, which can raise the risk of iron and zinc deficiencies. Avoid them if you can, or soak, sprout, or ferment them to reduce or eliminate the phytic acid.

REST

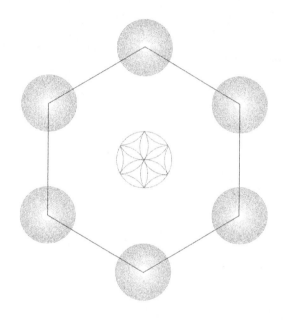

CHAPTER THREE

"I think many individuals in society feel uncomfortable about the idea of genetically modified embryos or even genetically modified food. But by choosing to get insufficient sleep, we may be forced to accept that we are performing a similar genetic modifying experiment on ourselves. And if we don't let our children get the sleep they so desperately need, we may be inflicting a similar genetic engineering experiment on them as well."

Professor Matthew Walker, Director of UC Berkeley's Sleep and Neuroimaging Lab

"I'LL SLEEP WHEN I'm dead."

I have heard this said a thousand times from a thousand of my Type-A friends, colleagues, and clients. Sleep is a luxury they couldn't afford. Or worse, that sleep is a non-essential in the modern world. It may have been a biological precaution for cavemen, a physical imperative to keep them safe in the dark nights of the past, but we've outgrown that. We have electricity and artificial light and we don't need to worry about a saber-toothed tiger dragging us away from our tribe if we take a walk in the middle of the night.

How many people did I know who *swore* they only needed five hours of sleep per night? Scientific research proves that to be a dangerous frame of mind. I get it because that used to be me: I had lived the mantra my whole life. I worked hard. I played hard. I'd take a nice long dirt nap when I died. Until then, I was busy!

Maybe you're different. Maybe you get eight hours of sleep every night and have educated yourself on the science of sleep. If so, you can skip this chapter. But that's probably not you. Statistically speaking, you likely don't get enough sleep. In fact, in the industrialized world today, one out of every two adults is trying to survive on six hours of sleep or less per night. Are you one of them?

Do you try to get by on six hours per night during the week then try to "catch up" on weekends? (Hint: that doesn't work!) Or maybe you've convinced yourself that you just don't need eight hours of sleep per night. You're the exception to the rule. One of the hallmarks of sleep deprivation is an impaired subjective appraisal of your own performance levels. Like a drunk at the bar who thinks he's okay to drive, people with sleep deprivation overestimate how well they are doing.

Like pretty much every other pillar in this book, I gained an appreciation for sleep through pain. As Paul Chek says, "Pain can be a great teacher." Pain can help make you aware of imbalances in your life. Drugs and alcohol caused deep physical and emotional pain earlier in my life, but I had found peace and balance in mind/body/spirit through nutrition, exercise, meditation, and strong personal relationships. The same would be true about sleep.

Now I was in my 40s and things were going great. I was eating healthy and taking care of myself. My acting career was thriving. I was married and had just had my first child. My life was busy, and sleep was not a priority. And then I hit a brick wall.

Many of the things I learned, my "pain teachers," have been through emotional manifestations. My temper gets short. I become angry. I lash out. I've become more and more aware of this as I grow older, and when I find myself getting angry and frustrated, I immediately begin examining my life to see where the stress lies.

4 am

The baby is crying. Again. Little Troy is 4 months old, and he is hungry.

In the broader scheme of things, I understand that I have it easier than my wife. My body isn't permanently altered by the birth of our son. Hormones aren't raging through my body like they are in hers. I don't have to suckle this baby at my breast to feed it (although, to be quite honest, I was sometimes curious – and maybe a little jealous – of that mother/baby bond).

But I am working harder than I ever had in my life. I have been up until 1:30 am editing video and posting to my YouTube channel. I am hustling to provide for my growing family. I change diapers, take on more of the household chores, rock the baby to sleep and rub my wife's aching feet and shoulders. When the baby cries, I often get up and bring him to his mother because I know how tired she is. I am building my legacy of being a humble, kind, and gentle man.

But on this night, I am bone tired. Completely exhausted. My body aches, and the cries of the baby seem like a bad dream. I just need to sleep.

"Can you get him," Uri moans, trying to rouse herself for the second feeding of the night (so far).

I pretend like I don't hear her. Maybe she'll take pity on me and let me sleep. "Troy!" She shakes me emphatically.

"What?" I croak, feeling the anger rise inside of me. "Little Troy is crying. Can you get him?"

"What's wrong with your legs?" I ask. Once a smartass, always a smartass. As soon as the words leave my mouth, I know that I have crossed a line, but let's just say I am not thinking clearly.

"They ache! That's what's the matter with them!"

Little Troy can hear us, but isn't sure if we can hear him, so he redoubles his efforts and turns the volume up a notch. The wailing rings in my ears.

"Goddammit, my legs ache too!" I scream. I am suddenly on my feet, anger rising up from my gut. I can taste it in the back of my throat like bile. I grab the alarm clock on my nightstand and throw it at the wall. It shatters to pieces.

My wife's eyes fill with tears as she hustles out of bed to scoop up Little Troy.

What just happened? That is not me. I am not like that! I am not a violent person, and I hate myself for scaring my wife like that. My stomach churns with guilt and remorse.

When my wife can finally look me in the eyes again, I apologize sincerely. "I am sorry," I say. "I don't know what came over me."

"It's okay," she smiles. "We're both just really tired."

The baby is soon fast asleep, and Uri isn't far behind. I lie there beside her, listening to her breathing, but the adrenaline is still coursing through my veins. I need to learn more about sleep and how it affects my mood.

That was 10 years ago. Since then, I've read about sleep extensively and incorporated good sleep hygiene into my routine. I've experienced firsthand how getting enough sleep can improve the quality of my life, and I know this information can help you too.

The Science of Sleep

The 21st century has been a renaissance for sleep science. Advancements in imaging technologies and gene mapping have allowed researchers to take a much closer look at what happens in your brain and your body when you sleep, as well as understanding the ill effects that sleep deprivation can have. Let's take a closer look.

Circadian Rhythm

As above, so below. This natural law of correspondence is evident in plants and animals on earth. Trees furl and unfurl their leaves as the sun rises and falls. Flowers open and close their petals. Animals – including humans – wake and sleep in 24-hour cycles.

Derived from the Latin *circa*, meaning "approximately" and *diem*, meaning "day," circadian rhythms refer to any biological process that works on 24-hour cycles.

Life on earth is intimately and inextricably bound to the celestial realm. For humans, the rising and falling of the sun is a cornerstone of our existence, and sleep is the most obvious outward display of this relationship. Light and dark trigger physiological changes in our bodies that control our sleep patterns.

But science has also proven that our circadian sleep patterns are endogenous, which means they're built in. Experiments in caves and other laboratory settings have shown that our circadian rhythms persist even when we are removed from the sun. 3.5 billion years of evolution has literally stitched circadian rhythms into the fabric of life on earth.

Just as with oxygen, food, and water, sleep is essential to life. You literally cannot live without it. There are rare cases where people – because of some brain injury or illness – lose the ability to sleep. Unfortunately for them, they quickly descend into madness and death.

Most likely, you have the ability to sleep, and if you left your body alone, it would get adequate sleep. You'd wake feeling refreshed, your body and mind would stay healthy, and you'd live a longer and happier life.

Humans are the only animal species known to voluntarily deprive themselves of sleep. As I mentioned before, fully half of all people living in the industrialized world do so.

Education systems usually have early start times. Workers often rise before the sun to start their busy days. People who "burn the midnight oil" wear their self-imposed sleep deprivation like a badge of honor, while those who get sufficient sleep are considered "lazy." What madness!

Hundreds of scientific studies bear out the truth: Short sleep = short life.

Well, I want to live a long and healthy life, and I've come to realize just how vital sleep is to that goal. Let's take a closer look at how sleep works.

In general, sleep is broken into two types: REM and non-REM (NREM). REM sleep is named for the rapid eye movements observed during this phase of sleep, which is usually associated with dreams. EEG imaging reveals that REM brain activity is similar to that of the waking brain. There are also marked changes in breathing, body temperature, and circulation.

Have you ever had a dream where you were trying to move, but couldn't – almost as if you were paralyzed? Well, technically you *are* paralyzed during REM sleep. Researchers believe this is an evolutionary safety mechanism that keeps your body from acting out your dreams. To keep you safe, your body inhibits motor neurons from firing, resulting in an almost complete paralysis.

Heart rate, blood pressure, and breathing also quickly become irregular during REM sleep. Body temperature is not well regulated and becomes more sensitive to external temperatures. Researchers believe these changes are important for maintaining cardiovascular health.

Non-REM (or NREM) sleep, by contrast, exhibits little eye movement. Dreams are rare, and muscles are not paralyzed. EEG imaging of the brain shows a completely different neurological pattern than what is seen in waking or REM sleep states. These images show highly complex "spindles" of electromagnetic activity, which activate different parts of the brain at different wavelengths. NREM sleep has been linked to memory and learning.

Have you ever seen the Pixar film "Inside Out?" This coming-of-age story takes us inside the mind of a teenage girl (Riley) dealing with a life-changing move across the country.

The animation personifies her emotions (Joy, Fear, Anger, Disgust, and Sadness). It also beautifully illustrates how sleep facilitates learning and memory.

In terms of memory, the hippocampus can be thought of as a sort of inbox. In the Pixar movie, each new memory or experience of the day appears as a shiny, color-coded sphere (where each color represents a different emotion). All of the days' memories are stacked up in a sort of pneumatic tube. When Riley falls asleep, those memories are moved from short-term to long-term memory (from the hippocampus to the cortex).

Scientists believe this is what happens during NREM sleep. The sleep spindles activate different parts of the brain at different times, sorting out the memories and storing them for long-term retention.

Laboratory tests have proven that it is nearly impossible to form new memories without sleep. One such experiment wanted to challenge the education myth of "pulling an all-nighter" before a big exam. Two groups of healthy young people were selected. One group was given a full eight hours of sleep, while the others stayed awake all night. Both groups were asked to memorize new information.

The results speak for themselves: The sleep-deprived group scored 40% lower than the sleep group. In education, that is the difference between acing the exam and failing miserably. Brain scans showed that the hippocampus was virtually inactive in the sleep-deprived group.

Sleep Cycles

Every night, a healthy sleeper will move through a sleep cycle approximately every 90 minutes. You will typically go through four to five cycles each night. Below is a brief description of the typical sleep cycle.

Stage 1

This transitional phase occurs as you move from wakefulness to sleep. During this NREM state, you may still be aware of your surroundings. You may start to drift off, only to experience a falling sensation that suddenly wakes you up.

Stage 2

This NREM stage is marked by light sleep in which your heart rate gradually begins to slow, and your body temperature begins to drop. Brain waves slow, with occasional bursts of spindles. In healthy sleep cycles, approximately half your night will be spent in Stage 2.

Stages 3 and 4

These "deep sleep" stages are grouped together because they are both slow-wave sleep (SWS) cycles characterized by active spindles that alternate in wavelength. People in these deep sleep stages are difficult to wake, and if they are woken, they will probably appear disoriented. In addition to moving the days' memories from short-term to long-term memory, hormones are released to aid appetite control, and blood flow to the muscles restores oxygen and nutrients. Simply speaking, the mind rests, while the body is rejuvenated.

Stage 5

Stage 5 is the only stage in which you get REM sleep. In this stage, your body rests while your brain bursts with activity. Your body is paralyzed, your eyes dart back and forth, and you dream. REM sleep is typically shorter earlier in the night and becomes longer as your sleep progresses. Some research suggests that REM sleep and dreams are essential for your emotional wellbeing.

Sleep is Mother Nature's way of repairing you – mentally and physi-cally – from the wear and tear of your everyday life. If you let sleep take its natural course, your mind and body will get the best possible care. But if you don't, there can be some truly awful effects on your mind and body. I cannot possibly list them all, but here are some negative side effects of sleep deprivation.

Cardiac Health

How much sleep do you really need to miss before it gets dangerous? One hour. That's it. One hour of missed sleep can be deadly.

The *BMJ* (originally the *British Medical Journal*) published a study linking heart attacks and daylight savings time. This man-made biannual ritual affects more than 1.6 billion people worldwide. Hospitals reported a 24% spike in heart attacks in the spring, when the affected population loses an hour of sleep. Correspondingly, researchers found a 21% decrease in heart attacks in the fall, when we are given an extra hour of sleep.

It's shocking to think how such a small change in sleep for one night could have such deadly consequences. Have you missed an hour of sleep this week? More? You could literally be killing yourself!

Sexual Health

It's a fact that men who sleep five hours a night have significantly smaller testicles than those who sleep eight hours or more. Put me in the big ball club!

In addition, men who routinely sleep only five to six hours a night will have a level of testosterone of someone ten years older. That's right! Short sleep ages you as a man. Whether you're planning to have a family or just enjoy a healthy sex life, sleep is your friend.

Mental and Emotional Health

The amygdala is the part of the brain most closely associated with emotional reactions. Brain scans show that the amygdala becomes 60% more responsive in people who are sleep deprived. If you're not getting enough sleep, you may have sudden mood swings and impulsive behavior. You could lash out at your loved ones and smash your alarm clock (like I did) because you are not in full control of your emotions.

Numerous studies are finding significant links between sleep disruption and conditions such as depression, anxiety, PTSD, schizophrenia, and suicide. In fact, there is not a single psychiatric condition in which sleep is normal. Whether that means the condition disrupts sleep, or disrupted sleep causes the condition is unclear, but sleep and mental health are inextricably linked.

Aging and Dementia

Sleep deprivation is also linked to cognitive decline, memory decline, and Alzheimer's disease. We know from imaging that the very structure and vasculature of the brain are altered as we age. We also know that sleep can speed up or slow down these processes.

Metabolism

Disruption of sleep can have a huge negative impact on your metabolic system. For instance, if you miss only one hour of sleep per night for one week, your blood sugar levels can rise to a pre-diabetic level. A 15-year longitudinal study found that people who self-reported getting six hours or less of sleep were twice as likely to develop diabetes.

Appetite

Your hypothalamus regulates the release of leptin and ghrelin, two hormones associated with appetite. Leptin is an appetite suppressant and is used to tell your body that it has enough fuel and to stop eating. Ghrelin, on the other hand, increases a sense of hunger and signals your body to end its fasting period and get more fuel. Studies have found links between sleep deprivation and levels of leptin and ghrelin in your body. In short, lack of sleep increases appetite by about 24%. Data also showed that sleep-deprived subjects had a preference for high-carb foods. If you're trying to lose weight, getting enough sleep can be one of the most effective things you can do.

Immune System

Your body produces cancer cells every day. When your immune system is working properly, the cancer cells are killed before they can start to form cancerous tumors. Sleep loss weakens your immune system and could allow the cancer cells to survive long enough to start growing in your body. Once that happens, lack of sleep becomes an accelerant for cancer growth. In fact, the link between lack of sleep and cancer is so strong that the World Health Organization recently classified any form of nighttime shift work as a probable carcinogen.

DNA

Lack of sleep doesn't just disrupt your body systems; it can mess with the very fabric of your biology: your DNA. A study was conducted on young healthy adults that limited them to six hours of sleep for one week. Researchers then measured the activity in the gene activity profile compared to when those same individuals were getting eight hours of sleep per night for a week.

The data showed sleep deprivation distorted the activity of more than 700 genes. Half the genes – those related to numerous aspects of the immune system – had decreased activity.

The other half – those related to the promotion of tumors, chronic inflammation, and stress – was upregulated in their expression.

As Professor Matthew Walker of UC Berkley puts it:

"There is simply no aspect of your physiology that seems to be able to retreat at the sign of sleep deprivation and get away unscathed. It's almost like a broken water pipe in your home. Sleep loss will leak down into every nook and cranny of your biology, even tampering with the very DNA nucleic alphabet that spells out your daily health narrative.

Sleep is not an optional lifestyle luxury. Sleep is a non-negotiable biological necessity. It's a life support system. It is Mother Nature's best effort yet at contra-death. And the decimation of sleep throughout industrialized nations is having a catastrophic impact on our health, our wellness, and the safety and education of our children."

If you are in the 50% of the population that gets six hours or less sleep per night, I hope this has helped you understand the folly of your ways. You can eat organic, go to the gym every day, and do all the other healthy things you like, but if you're not getting enough sleep, you are undermining your own progress, and literally killing yourself. Once I adopted good sleep hygiene, everything improved. I felt better mentally and physically, my relationships were richer and less stressed, and I was able to perform better on every level.

So, what can you do to make sure you get enough sleep? Here are some tips for good sleep hygiene:

The National Sleep Foundation recommends that adults 26-64 get between 7 and 9 hours of sleep per night, and adults 65 and over get 7 to 8 hours of sleep. Each person is different, so you'll need to find the right amount of sleep for you. When you get enough sleep, you should wake feeling refreshed and not feel sleepy during the day.

When to Sleep

The best way to keep your circadian rhythms intact is to go to bed and wake up at the same time each day. This can be difficult for some people, especially on the weekends. If you've missed sleep during the week, you may feel like sleeping in on the weekends to catch up, but this only continues to disrupt your circadian rhythms. Find a schedule and stick to it every day.

You've probably also noticed that some people are "morning people" and others are "night owls." This is known as your chronotype. On average, sleeping from 10:00 pm to 6:00 am is ideal, but depending on your chronotype, you may naturally prefer to go to sleep earlier or later. Respect your chronotype and your circadian rhythm and find a schedule that is right for you.

Light and Sleep

As we discussed earlier in this chapter, we are biologically wired to wake when it is light out and sleep when it is dark. In the modern world, however, these circadian rhythms can be disrupted by electric lights and LED displays. They alter our brain chemistry and make natural sleep more difficult. At the end of the day, you need to let your mind wind down and prepare for sleep. Bombarding your eyes with artificial light is a problem, as the blue light spectrum of computer monitors, tablets, and cell phones has been shown to suppress the secretion of melatonin – a hormone that is important in sleep.

Eliminating exposure to blue light one to two hours before bedtime is ideal. Many new phones and tablets have blue blocker technology, so check your devices to see if you can turn off the blue light spectrum. If not, or if you are watching TV, try blue blocker glasses.

Try to use salt lamps, candles, and/or nightlights to decrease your light exposure, and make sure your bedroom is dark. Remove bright lights (including bright alarm clocks) and use curtains, shades, or even a sleeping mask to help. If you get up at night to go to the bathroom, don't turn the lights on. Use a nightlight to find your way safely.

Temperature

Temperature plays a critical role in sleep. If your body is too warm, it will be hard for you to fall asleep. Exercising can raise your core temperature, and studies have found those who exercise in the morning sleep better than those who exercise at night. Taking a cool bath or shower before bed and keeping your bedroom cool can also help you fall asleep faster and get better quality sleep.

Diet

Eating a lot of food at night, especially sugar, can disrupt your sleep patterns. You should avoid eating large meals within three hours of sleep and stay away from sugar and refined carbohydrates.

Caffeine

Caffeine is the second most traded commodity on earth (behind oil) and has found its way into the lives of most adults and even children. When it comes to sleep, caffeine can be a true enemy. Caffeine can affect your sleep up to 12 hours after you've ingested it. If you do drink caffeine, try to limit it to the morning hours and avoid it later in the day. Or, better yet, remove it from your diet entirely!

Alcohol and Marijuana

People often say that alcohol and/or marijuana help relax them at night and put them to sleep. While on the surface, this might seem plausible, both substances are counterproductive to quality sleep.

Research shows both have a negative effect on REM sleep, so it's best to avoid them for the best possible sleep.

Sleeping Pills

Sleeping pills can be downright dangerous and should be avoided except in extreme cases. They have been linked to cancer and other serious illnesses, as well as mood disorders, accidental deaths, and suicides. Yet for all the downsides, sleeping pills have very few (if any) benefits. These hypnotic drugs essentially knock out the cortex, or consciousness, but they disrupt the natural NREM and REM cycles of healthy sleep. Stay away from them!

Stress

Stress is a killer, literally. It affects your mood, your thoughts, your metabolism, your immune system, and your sleep. Conversely, sleep can be one of the best antidotes to stress. Adopt relaxing nighttime rituals to prepare yourself for a good night's sleep.

Meditate. Take a bath. Have a cup of caffeine-free herbal tea. Take your dog for a walk. Snuggle. Read a book (a real book, not an eBook). Whatever it is that makes you feel calm and peaceful, do it.

Naps

If you do have sleep deficits, the best thing to do is make them up with naps. But be careful! Sleeping for more than 20 minutes at a time during the day can be counterproductive and make it harder for you to fall asleep at night.

By practicing good sleep hygiene, you can restore your natural circadian rhythm, enjoy a good night's sleep, and wake feeling refreshed. You'll boost your immune system, strengthen your heart, regulate your mood, and balance your hormones. You'll find balance. Homeostasis.

And oh, what dreams may come!

Getting enough sleep is essential for good health, yet nearly half of all adults in the industrialized world try to survive on six hours of sleep per night or less. Here are some good sleep hygiene tips to help you build your Rest Pillar:

1. **Honor your circadian rhythms** – go to bed and get up at the same time each day (even on the weekends).

2. **Artificial light** – electronic devices and artificial light can disrupt your sleep patterns. Use these strategies to get the best sleep possible:

   a. Eliminate exposure to blue light 1-2 hours before bedtime.

   b. Use blue blocker technology on newer phones and tablets.

   c. Use blue blocker glasses for older phones/tablets or for watching TV.

   d. Remove bright lights (including alarm clocks and other electronic devices) from your bedroom.

   e. Use salt lamps, candles, and/or nightlights at night.

3. **Temperature** – high body temperature can equal poor sleep. Keep your bedroom cool and avoid exercise too close to bedtime. A cool bath or shower can help reduce your core temperature and produce higher-quality sleep.

4. **Diet** – avoid a lot of food, especially sugar, at night.

5. **Caffeine** – can stay in your system for up to 10 hours. Limit your caffeine intake to the mornings, or better yet remove it from your diet completely.

6. **Alcohol and marijuana** – have a negative impact on REM sleep and should be avoided.

7. **Sleeping pills** – can be downright dangerous. Avoid them except in extreme cases.

8. **Stress** – can disrupt your sleep. Adopt relaxing nighttime rituals to prepare for a good night's sleep. Do whatever makes you feel calm and peaceful.

9. **Naps** – If you are still tired during the day, short naps can be rejuvenating. Remember to limit them to 20 minutes – otherwise, you could have trouble falling asleep at night.

MOVEMENT

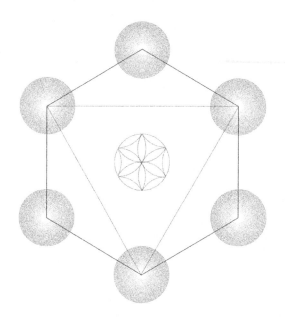

CHAPTER FOUR

"Nothing happens until something moves."

Albert Einstein

A S A CHILD, I was blessed to have the experience of living in nature. We lived on a small lake in rural Connecticut and also in Marin County, California, just north of San Francisco. I had a lot of freedom to roam the woods by myself unsupervised. In many ways, I remember it as an idyllic childhood.

By many standards, my childhood was not idyllic. I remember a time my friends and I were all going to my friend Tommy's house for his 12th birthday. They had a pool, and we were going to hang out all weekend swimming, playing Atari, and looking at some imported French porno mags that Anthony found in his uncle's basement.

"You need to learn to fend for yourself," my stepfather, Jack, said when I asked for a ride. "I can't ride my bike there. It's 15 miles away," I groused. "Can't you drive me?"

"Have you seen the price of gas these days?" he said, cracking open another beer. I looked at my mom for help, but she just shrugged her shoulders.

"What the hell am I supposed to do?" I asked.

My stepfather raised his thumb and pointed at it. "You know what that is?" "A thumb?" I said, not sure where this was going.

He held his thumb out, pantomiming the hitchhiking gesture. "You're smarter than you look, Troy. Why don't you go outside and try it out? I am sure you'll get a ride."

It took me all afternoon to cover the 15 miles to Tommy's house, but I got there eventually. I never asked my stepfather for a ride again, which he probably considered a great success and a life lesson learned.

Jack also beat me. He worked the graveyard shift at a nearby factory and complained all the time about the toxic crap they had him working with. The hours were long, the pay was shitty, and the chronic lack of sleep made him a bear to be around. He took his frustrations out on me and my brother Shawn.

One day, in a fit of rage, he told me to pack my things. I stuffed what few possessions I owned into two pillowcases and put them on the porch. I was in the kitchen saying goodbye to my mom, but she wasn't taking it too seriously. We'd had these kinds of talks a hundred times before, and I hadn't left yet.

Jack went out onto the porch for a smoke and tripped over my stuff. That really set him off. Why did I leave all my shit on the porch? I probably did it to trip him. He took off his belt, and I could tell by the color of his face that this day's beating would be worse than normal.

Unfortunately, that was a pretty typical Sunday.

By the time I was a teenager, Jack got fed up with factory life and started dealing pot. Things got a little better for a short while. The beatings became less frequent and less severe. My mom got a new car. But then he got busted by the FBI, and everything turned to shit. The beatings got worse, and before I knew it, the family broke up. By the age of 14, I was on my own. I stayed at friends' houses. I slept in their basements or on their couches when I could. I bounced around from school to school and managed to get kicked out of most of them.

I scrounged food when I could, but I went to bed hungry more times than I can count. Having never had a real job, I didn't know how to make money. One summer, I built a house for $2/hour plus room and board. But by the time I was 17, I dreamed of getting my own car, and I needed cash.

I hitchhiked into San Francisco, then walked up to Haight-Ashbury to score some acid. I figured I could double my money, and it was a hell of a lot easier than working construction. I was an entrepreneur.

I told Tommy and Carl, and soon everyone knew where to get their LSD. My friends scored at cost, and that asshole Erik P. and his jerk buddies paid through the nose for their tabs.

I had a girlfriend named Tina at the time, and her father really hated me. Go figure. I stopped going over to Tina's house because her dad gave me a hard time every time he saw me. But we still hooked up. There was always a party somewhere, or a bunch of us would get together in the park and hang out. That burned her old man up.

Tina had a couple of cousins in the area: Danny and Donna. They were nice, but not the sharpest tools in the shed. I am not sure how it all went down, but one of them let it slip to their mom that I was dealing acid. Their mom called Tina's dad, and he called the cops.

Tina's dad seemed to have some kind of pull somewhere, because they started an investigation. I learned after the fact that they followed me for three days. It amazes me to think that with all the stuff going down around there at the time, they had the time to trail me.

They were trying to catch me in the act of selling, but they never did. Not because I was too clever for them, but because I had just run out of supply. I guess they just got tired of waiting. One day as I was on my way to breakfast, they pulled me over and searched me. I had just scored the night before and so they popped me with a sheet of acid in my wallet. 100 hits.

Busted.

In hindsight, I was pretty lucky. Four months later and I would have been an adult. That probably would have meant years behind bars. But since I was underage, I ended up as a ward of the state and was sent to juvenile detention.

Juvie wasn't bad. I got three squares a day and didn't have any bills to pay. They had a weight room and a library, so I could pump iron and read as much as I wanted.

About a week after I got busted, I had a court date. My probation officer took me to the courthouse in handcuffs, but when we got there he took them off and went to talk to the court officials about something. That's when I ran into my friend Kenny.

"Kenny," I said, giving him a high five. "What are you doing here?"

"Remember that 350-cubic-inch engine my dad and I dropped in mom's Corvette last month?" asked Kenny, smiling. Not really. Kenny and his dad were total gearheads and always talking torque and lift and gapping the plugs, but that wasn't my thing. I just nodded my head.

"Well, I wanted to try it out, but she wouldn't let me. So I rolled it down the driveway when she was asleep and took it for a spin," he bragged. "I was roasting tires in the Kmart parking lot when the cops busted me." He said it like he'd just won a medal at state or something.

"Hey, can I stay at your house for a while?"

"Let me ask," he said, looking around the room for his mom. We spotted her in the back, chatting with an elderly acupuncturist with a heavy Chinese accent.

"Hey mom, can Troy stay over at our house for a while?" Kenny asked.

"Sure thing, honey," she said without missing a beat. I don't know if she was just oblivious or what, but it didn't seem to strike her as odd at all that I was asking this question at the courthouse. Kenny was an only child and spoiled rotten, so he got pretty much anything he wanted.

The probation officer was still talking to someone, so I slipped out a side door and found my way down a back stairwell to the alley. I snuck around the perimeter of the building, then took off running. So long, suckers!

I made it over to another friend's house, and he called Kenny to come pick me up. Kenny had his own wheels, of course, and came over later that night. "The cops are asking around for you," he said, a bit of envy in his voice. "You better lay low for a while."

Kenny took me past Tina's house. There was a cop car in the driveway, so we parked a few blocks away. I crept up from the back.

"Oh my God, what did you do?" Tina asked through the screen. I had climbed a tree next to her second-story bedroom window and threw pebbles and the glass until she noticed me.

"I skipped out," I told her.

"Well, they're pretty mad, Troy. I think you're in a lot of trouble." "Nothing I can't handle," I said, trying to sound tough.

"What are you going to do now?" she asked.

"I'm thinking about heading east. Going to see my grandma in Connecticut."

"That's a good idea," she said. She blew me a kiss, and I climbed down and ran back to Kenny's car.

"You still wanna sleep at my house?" he asked.

"Nah. They've probably got your place staked out. Better take me to the Greyhound station."

Kenny dropped me off and gave me all the money in his wallet: $27. That gave me almost $200. I bought a one-way ticket, got a sandwich from the vending machine, and had enough left over for three or four meals if I skimped. Who says you can't outrun the long arm of the law!

Two days later, we rolled into Cheyenne, WY. The guy next to me had been farting for the last two hundred miles and the bus had a thick traveler's funk. I needed to stretch my legs and take a leak. But as we pulled up to the station, I saw a bunch of cop cars and knew the jig was up.

I spent ten days in a private cell in Cheyenne before the extradition paperwork came through. They sent me back to California, where I appeared in front of a judge. This time, when my probation officer took off the cuffs, he never took his eyes off of me.

I got off pretty easy – the judge gave me 4 ½ months in juvenile detention.

"You'll be 18 years old when you get out, Mr. Casey," he lectured. "If you try any of these tricks again, the next judge will not be so lenient. My advice to you is to use your time in juvenile detention to examine your life and think about what you want to do with it. It really is up to you."

I am not sure if the judge knew it, but his words resonated. I wanted to make something of my life, and I could see how hard that would be from behind bars. I never wanted to have this experience again, so I set my mind and my body to work.

The library turned out to be pretty decent. I didn't want to fall behind in school, so I read and studied for hours every day. I read about history and science. I read Shakespeare and Ayn Rand. I improved my vocabulary and learned about world religions. I've always had a curious mind, and I was free to read whatever interested me. And everything interested me.

I spent a lot of my time in the weight room too, and I dove into working out with gusto. I trained there with other guys and they helped push me along. It was incredible how much muscle mass I gained in such a short time. I pumped up fast. But even more than just looking ripped, what really grabbed me was how much better I felt after I worked out. Pumping iron relaxed me. I wasn't as angry, and I didn't have as many negative thoughts zipping around my head all day. Moving my body made me feel better. I got an adrenaline high that was undeniable.

On days when I didn't work out, I felt more lethargic and my mood was darker. I could get down on myself and think terrible thoughts. As long as I kept my body moving, I was alright. I didn't realize it at the time, but I was beginning awakening to my mind/body connection. It would be years before I could articulate it, but I was beginning to understand that movement was essential to my health (both mentally and physically).

In the years since then, I have learned again and again that the mind is an embodied process. I've learned that it is impossible to separate your emotional health and your physical health. I have learned that your issues really do store in your tissues.

In the rest of this chapter, I am going to share what I have learned about movement, and how those lessons helped me become *RippedAt50*. I hope you find this information helpful.

For much of my early adulthood, I had a career in modeling, so my intention was to look good for the camera. I wanted healthy hair and skin, six-pack abs, and sex appeal. As I moved from modeling to acting, I wanted those same things, but I took a much wider view. I wanted *functional* fitness. I wanted to live without pain and to move gracefully. I wanted to have energy to play with my kids, ride my bike, or take long hikes. I wanted to dance all night and feel like a million bucks. I wanted to live a long and healthy life.

In my fifties, I am in the best shape of my life. I have been able to "master" The 9 Pillars, put all of the lessons I've learned together, and achieve my dreams. I use the word "master" in quotes here because as you will learn from reading this book, I am far from infallible, and I still make lots of mistakes. What I mean is that I've internalized the lessons in my life and continue to work very hard every day to live what I've learned as authentically as I can. I've seen the impact that each pillar has on my life. And I've witnessed the fact that when I finally put them all together, the results are astounding. No one is perfect, least of all me. But The 9 Pillars have served me well.

When it comes to creating a life that incorporates movement, the first and most important thing you need to do is be clear on your intention. Do you want to climb Mt. Everest, run the Boston marathon, or hike the Pacific Crest Trail? Do you want to be able to pick up your kids? Your grandkids? Your great-grandkids? Do you want to have a healthy sex life into your 90s? Whatever it is you desire, the first step to making it happen is to visualize it.

Top athletes do this. Highly successful entrepreneurs do this. It is a critical step that cannot be skipped. Imagine trying to drive from New York to Los Angeles without a roadmap or GPS. You might get there eventually, but it's going to take a lot longer and may take you in unintended – and unwanted – directions.

There are many different techniques for visualization, and you should find something that works for you. Athletes do "mental rehearsals," visualizing themselves throwing a curveball across the outside corner of the plate or taking every turn in a downhill slalom run. Others use meditation, affirmations, vision boards, journaling, or hypnosis.

Regardless of the technique, these steps activate the subconscious brain to begin solving the challenge needed to achieve the goal. By bringing these thoughts into existence, you give them form and substance as you move from dream to reality. They take on a gravity of their own, and you begin to attract the people and resources you need to succeed.

Providence rises up to meet you.

To paraphrase Napoleon Hill, from his seminal book *Think and Grow Rich,* whatever the mind can conceive and believe, the body can achieve.

Once your intention is set and your vision is clear, you can begin to achieve your goals. But before you begin to move, you should do your homework. Too many people think you need to be a "gym rat" to succeed. They dive in headlong without having a clue of what they are doing.

"I burned 1,300 calories!"

"Man, you should have seen me sweat." "No pain, no gain."

That's how people get hurt. And I am not talking about the muscle soreness that can come with a good workout. I am talking about debilitating injuries that can take months or years to heal.

If you don't know what you're doing, you should consult a professional. Stay away from the hacks and meatheads out there who can do more harm than good. My personal favorite is Paul Chek. His book

How to Eat, Move, and Be Healthy is considered by many to be the bible on movement and nutrition.

I started watching Paul's videos in 2008. His information was the most comprehensive presentation on nutrition that I had ever seen anywhere. He was not discussing macronutrients, carbs, fat, and protein – he was talking about the microbes in the soil and the cosmic energy that is collected by the piezoelectric rocks in the earth! He wasn't daunted by the fact that some considered this information "airy-fairy stuff." So-called experts had ignored and dismissed some of the concepts he was teaching, but now hard science was proving those "experts" wrong. Paul was the greatest teacher I could find, and I owe him my deepest gratitude, love, and respect.

After following his work for a few years, I began to turn many others on to him. One of my friends was making a film on epigenetics and healing the body by taking responsibility for everything in your life. He asked me to go to San Diego to help him film pickups for inter- views he had done previously. Paul Chek was on the list. After we filmed the pickups, I asked Paul if I could interview him for Certified Health Nut, and the rest is history. We've been friends ever since.

In 2011, I was asked by Paul and Penny Chek to film and interview practitioners and coaches at the C.H.E.K. Conference, a seminar and gathering of C.H.E.K.-educated professionals in the healing arts and sports fitness world. After reading his books and following him on the Internet, I finally got to meet him in person. I got a personal invitation to go to his house. I was honored.

The twenty-five or so practitioners I interviewed all had amazing posture and bodies that were like gorillas in the wild: erect, muscular, ripped, clear-headed, and coherent. They exuded a confidence of KNOWING sans pretense. This was a welcome respite after all the egos and attitudes I experienced in LA. To have this many humble high-achievers in one room was unprecedented in my experience. Never before had I met a group of people who literally embodied the large database of information. Knowledge is one thing.

Experience is another. These people were living their knowledge authentically. I realized how powerful the C.H.E.K. community was and saw its potential in transforming the world. As a sapiosexual (one who gets off on the intelligent use and application of knowledge), I was blown away at the level of consciousness on display.

Over the next two years, I enrolled in as many C.H.E.K. Institute classes as I could, including the entire Holistic Lifestyle Coaching series. What I got was a world-class education on how the human body functions, governed by the natural law of the universe. But for me and many of my colleagues, it is not about the information. It is the *application* of the information to one's own lifestyle that has any ballast in reality. To apply information for optimization of one's own biology, physiology, and psychology with the subsequent success in the realm of holistic health was a joy to witness. In my experience, most "healthy people" are not fit, most "fit people" are not healthy, and most "spiritual people" are neither healthy nor fit. So I found great comfort being amongst people who endeavored to achieve a higher level of human development.

Paul is one of, if not THE, best strength and conditioning coaches in the world. He's worked with more medically-retired athletes than anyone else on the face of the planet. He's huge in the world of rehabilitation: Danny Way, the famous skateboarder; Robbie Maddison, the modern-day Evel Knievel; Ryan Hughes, motocross champion; Laird Hamilton, the biggest surfing legend of our time. Paul has helped them all.

Danny Way broke his neck back in '94. Doctors said he'd never walk again. Four months later, the dude walked out of Paul's office and has been setting world records ever since.

Robbie Maddison almost punctured his aorta. Doctors told him he'd never ride a motorcycle again, and some thought he wouldn't survive. Two weeks later, Paul led him through some Qigong breathing exercises, his rib popped out, and Robbie jumped Caesar's Palace the next year.

Laird Hamilton didn't wait until he was hurt. He went to Paul proactively, looking for ways to live more optimally. Laird has a 10-point plan to live forever, and if anyone can help him figure it out, it's Paul.

Paul is also credited with ushering in the Swiss Ball and all the functional fitness we see in gyms today. When I was growing up, weightlifting was all about machines. Paul introduced kettlebells as well as lifting and balancing on Swiss balls and really thinking about the core. And then, just because he's Paul, he became a pioneer in thinking about how the gut microbiome is related to core functionality. You see, his wife studied biochemical anthropology at Cambridge, and he became fascinated with Paleo diets and the gut microbiome. And the kicker is...he was self-taught. He's a ninth-grade dropout who read thousands of books and has a fantastic and curious mind.

Paul founded the C.H.E.K (Corrective Holistic Exercise Kinesiology) Institute in California as a focal point for the education of elite health and exercise professionals. The C.H.E.K. Institute runs advanced certification programs and provides numerous training videos and courses to students worldwide. If you can work with Paul or one of his certified trainers, you are in good hands.

They start with a comprehensive set of assessment techniques to determine your current state of health and fitness, then tailor programs to meet your goals and lifestyle. I learned so much from him about the relationships between the musculoskeletal system and the glands, organs, posture, and breathing. Working with Paul was transformative. And believe me, once you've worked with him, it becomes easy to spot "trainers" who are faking it. If there is a trainer at your gym, or one in your area that you want to work with, just do your research and make sure you are working with a professional who has your best interest at heart. Anyone who puts you into a high-intensity workout without first assessing you or asking about your goals is not someone you should be working with (let alone paying).

When it comes to being physically active, if you are a true do-it-yourselfer, don't worry. You don't have to hire anyone or work with a trainer. I urge you to do an honest assessment of your functional fitness, then work slowly to build up strength and core stability. Remember that movement is part of a holistic approach to fitness that includes all the other pillars. They are interrelated and cannot be addressed by themselves.

Walking

My favorite movement is walking. It's true! I've gone years without seeing the inside of a gym and have kept myself lean and trim simply by walking. I remember early on in my modeling career I was living in Miami Beach, hanging out and partying all the time. I was spending a lot of time with Kim, a beautiful young model from Tennessee. She was new to the scene, but I could tell she'd go far. She was full of life, and a lot of fun to be with.

After a few months in Miami Beach, she left for New York to kick her career into high gear. I went to the city a few months later for a shoot and met her as she came out of her fourth meeting of the day. She looked amazing! She had trimmed down and toned up. She was practically glowing.

"My God, girl! What have you been doing?"

"Nothing!" she laughed, twirling to show off her sleek body. "Just walking." She took my elbow, and we started to stroll down W. 86th toward Central Park. It was a beautiful spring day in New York, and the streets were bustling.

"I've been so busy here, Troy," she beamed. "I've done eight shoots and probably a hundred interviews since I got here. And I walk *everywhere*. Seriously, I am probably walking 8 to 10 miles a day, and I feel great."

I'd noticed that in places like New York, Milan, and Tokyo, people do tend to walk everywhere. And not the stiff, unbalanced kind of walking you see so much of these days (overweight, stressed out, misaligned). A lot of people look like they're in pain with every step. But here, on this glorious afternoon in Central Park, bodies were moving gracefully. Purposefully. Happily.

We stopped on the lawn between the Natural History Museum and the Met and took off our shoes. Looking around, I could see dozens of people doing the same in ones and twos, and a group of about 20 doing Tai Chi over by Turtle Pond. I was intrigued.

Years later, I would attend a workshop by the great Taoist Master Mantak Chia. Master Chia inherited the complete Taoist internal spiritual cultivation system from his master, Yi Eng, and has spent his life teaching it to others. Coming from the Dragon's Gate sect of the Quanzhen (Complete Perfection) school of Taoism, Master Chia believes that it is the birthright of all humans to develop states of inner experience and consciousness. He emphasizes that this should be accessible to everyone without the superfluous rituals.

Master Chia teaches that the earth has a negative redux potential which will take out the positively charged toxins and also negative emotions. I know he speaks the truth.

Frolicking in the sun that afternoon, digging my toes into the broad green blades of grass, I felt all the negative emotions in my gut run to ground. I couldn't help but laugh out loud. And why not? Life is beautiful!

Walking is the perfect expression of how the human body was meant to move through time and space. Kim's lithe figure and balanced gait embodied the ideal portrait of ourselves as we're meant to be. We spent hours in the park, strolling from one end to the other, catching up on old times. Kim was also comfortable with silence, so for a time, we just walked side by side in a movement meditation that rejuvenated our bodies and calmed our minds.

In addition to moving oxygen and nutrients to every part of the body, walking also moves the lymph. Part of circulation, your lymphatic system moves vital fluids through the body. But unlike the circulatory system, it isn't a closed system. Every day, your body processes about 20 liters of blood through a capillary filtration system – separating plasma from blood cells. Approximately 17 liters of the filtered plasma returns to the body through the blood vessels, while the other 3 return via the lymphatic system. Your lymph nodes, together with your spleen and thymus, aid your immune system and support your digestive system.

Movement is also critical for a healthy autonomic nervous system – that involuntary system that unconsciously controls your heart, lungs, and digestive system. The sympathetic nervous system (SMS) and the parasympathetic nervous system (PSNS) work together, acting as a sort of on/off switch for many of your body's basic responses. In other words, one system may be responsible for causing a reaction while the other system is responsible for inhibiting that same reaction.

The sympathetic nervous system (SMS) is sometimes called the "fight-or-flight" system. If you perceive threat or danger, the SMS floods your body with neurotransmitters such as adrenaline. This involuntary response to threat is an important survival mechanism that kept our distant ancestors from being eaten in the jungle.

The parasympathetic nervous system (PSNS) is sometimes called the "rest-and-digest" or "feed-and-breed" system. After our ancestors escaped the jungle cat, their PSNS used different neurotransmitters, like acetylcholine, to bring their bodies back to a state of rest. The PSNS oversees bodily functions like digestion, urination, defecation, and sexual arousal.

But in the concrete jungle we live in today, the stressors that activate our fight-or-flight response are very different. Financial pressures. Deadlines at work. Environmental pollution. Contaminated food and water sources. These stressors can keep us in a constant state of alertness. A stressed mind is a stressed body. And a stressed body is an unhealthy body.

Cortisol and insulin are two primary hormonal pathways that must be in balance for optimal health. Produced by the adrenal gland (and in other tissues in lower quantities) cortisol is part of our natural diurnal cycle. When the sun rises, cortisol helps wake the body up. In the early stages of fasting, cortisol activates anti-stress and anti-inflammatory pathways. Later in fasting, cortisol helps the liver take up glucose and store it as fat.

Mother Nature has provided a beautiful and elegant banking system for our bodies, allowing us to deposit and withdraw energy and avoid starvation.

Under stressful conditions, cortisol can tap into these protein deposits via glucogenesis, which is helpful in a fight-or-flight response to give you a sudden burst of energy. But when your body is exposed to chronically elevated cortisol levels, glucose (or blood sugar) rises. Your body naturally releases insulin, which the cells of your body need to convert the glucose into energy. Over time, your cells can become insulin-resistant, preventing them from using the glucose effectively. To counteract the rising blood sugar level, your body releases more cortisol, and a vicious cycle begins.

Each of the 9 Pillars is essential for balance. If one pillar is out of balance, the whole structure is out of balance. On the one hand, it is a good thing that these pillars are interconnected. If one pillar is weakened, others can compensate. Life is a dynamic system, and adaptability is essential to survival. On the other hand, an imbalance in any one pillar affects all of the others. They are interrelated by design and cannot be separated. And each stressor can become a multiplier, affecting all of your pillars.

Being able to recognize your stressors and having solid strategies and tactics for counterbalancing their effects will help you achieve and maintain balance.

Movement is one of the best tools you have in your toolkit. As my grandma used to say, "Use it or lose it." Learn to use the tool of movement. Become a master carpenter of your body and your mind through the intelligent use of this precious gift we have been graced with.

Walking barefoot in the grass or in the water at the beach is one of my favorite things in life. Going deep into the woods energizes my body, mind, and spirit. Hiking, camping, and being in the wild can feel like a healing health retreat.

A stressed mind is a stressed body, and a stressed body is a stressed mind. This is a biological fact that you cannot escape. I've quantified and cataloged the stressors that disrupt the systems of your body and prevent homeostasis below.

Here are the **7 Factors of Stress:**

1. Physical
2. Digital Communications
3. Psychic
4. Nutritional
5. Thermal
6. Electromagnetic Fields (EMF) and Electromagnetic Radiation (EMR)
7. Chemical

Let's take a look at each one.

Physical Stress

Movement can be medicine. But like everything, it has a time and place. If you are tired, weak, overworked, or physically exhausted, you could be doing more harm than good by pushing your body.

An honest assessment of your energy levels on a daily (or even an hourly) basis will help you manage this form of stress. For example, if you feel tired or sore from the previous day's workout, take inventory to see if you have the proper energy to do the work you intend to do. Rest or take a nap if you can. If you are continuously running into this stress, make sure that you are using your time off from work to rest, rejuvenate, or meditate. You can rotate working out with walking, Qigong, Tai Chi, gentle stretching, or restorative yoga.

Don't buy into the "no pain, no gain" myth. Let your body rest when it needs to rest.

Even though you release endorphins and other feel-good chemicals during strenuous exercise, you run the risk of breaking your body down with cortisol and other stress hormones in the process. Your body can eventually become overwhelmed, which can result in burnout, injuries, or inability to recover from muscle soreness. Be honest with how you feel physically. Take it easy on days when you don't have the energy and "go big" on the days you do!

Digital Communication Stress

The advent of the Internet, mobile phones, and digital devices seems to have occurred in the blink of an eye. We live in a "connected" world with 24-hour news cycles and non-stop social media buzz. Technology giants are using AI to design ever more addictive ways to keep us interacting with our devices and engaging in more and more digital communication. They say the average teenager spends more time on a cell phone than sleeping. In 2018, the *Journal of the American Medical Association* recognized a new mental illness classified on the obsessive-compulsive spectrum called "Snapchat Dysmorphia."

You see, the picture-sharing social media site with its "fun" photo filters has been driving more and more teenagers to plastic surgeons in a quest to look more like their social media selves.

We are the guinea pigs in a grand new technological experiment, and no one knows the full impact that these devices and digital communications are having on our brains and our health. But a growing body of evidence is starting to outline the negative impacts.

Digital communication is a huge part of our daily lives, and I am not suggesting the path to optimal health means giving up technology. But you need to be mindful of how you use this technology, and guard yourself against technology using you.

Being always connected – always "on" – is known to raise stress levels and have a negative impact on your mental, physical, and emotional health. I use an app to monitor my screen time, and I set daily and weekly limits for my kids and myself. We have implemented a strict "no devices" rule around the dinner table. I use blue blocker technology on my phone to reduce blue light exposure later in the day, and I never keep a phone, computer, or any other messaging device in my bedroom at night.

Being mindful of how much digital communication you consume can help to reduce stress.

Psychic Stress

We all know hanging out with good friends can make us feel wonderful. Some friends just make us laugh, and we can feel the stress of the day melt away. The opposite is also true, as other people can have a draining effect; their negative energy seems to always bring us down.

The bottom line is that these energies all take a toll on our psyche. I practice ways to draw healthy boundaries and know how to balance and release these types of energies. I try to be aware of who I am hanging out with, and constantly ask myself, "Is this person making me feel good or bad?" If they make me feel bad, I try to limit my time with them, so they don't rob me of my positive energy.

Nutritional Stress

Unfortunately, too many people suffer nutritional stress. They eat commercial food that is not conducive to human consumption or matched to their own biochemistry. The foods cause inflammation, raise blood sugar levels, compromise the immune system, and stress all of our body's systems.

As we talked about before, just eat real food! Eat food that makes you feel satisfied, clean, clear, and strong. Eating regularly will help keep your blood sugar balanced, which is in direct correlation to insulin, a part of the primary hormonal pathways (cortisol, adrenaline, and insulin). These hormones are critical for balance and health. Keeping them as close to homeostasis as possible will keep you looking and feeling your best. Eat when you are hungry and try to take in a good balance of fats, carbohydrates, and protein. This will help the fuel metabolize and support your biochemistry. It's best for you as an individual to feel your way through what your body requires on any given day instead of listening to this diet paradigm or that famous person. It may work for them at a certain period in their life, but it may not work for you ever. Eat real, farmer direct, organic, grass-fed, free-range, whole foods. Eat what you like or are attracted to, pay attention to what digests well, rotate different foods, and practice fasting.

Thermal Stress

We are warm-blooded creatures, which means that our bodies are designed to operate at a steady temperature. Mother Nature has equipped us with ingenious ways to heat and cool ourselves to operate optimally. But in the modern world, we are often moving in and out of artificial environments that subject our bodies to huge temperature swings, thus subjecting us to thermal stress.

Being too cold can restrict blood circulation and energy flow. It can be a low-level stress that contracts muscles and eventually exhausts the immune system. Overheating our bodies can overwhelm our systems too.

By subjecting our bodies to thermal stress, forcing our systems to work harder to maintain a constant temperature, we divert energy that could be used by our digestive or immune systems.

Thermal stress affects our energy levels and our moods. The more we can understand and manage our energy through the day, the more balanced, healthy, and energized we can stay. Thermal stress from artificial and natural environments can be subtle, but they can also be abrupt or even drastic. Pay attention and have layers available, along with different hats, beanies for the cold, and wide brim or baseball hats for the sun!

EMF/EMR

Electromagnetic Fields (EMF) and Electromagnetic Radiation (EMR) may be some of the biggest unseen stressors in our modern world. Nikola Tesla had more inventions than Thomas Edison. He invented the 60Hz cycle that our electricity runs on. Five years after its use was in full effect, he discovered it was far from optimal for human beings because of the impact it had on our electrical field. When this was brought up to the industrialists, they said it would be too expensive to change the technology.

The result is that for the last 100 years or so, we have been using this form of "dirty" electricity. Take a break from this by turning off the breakers in your house. It feels like you are in the woods: clean, clear, and peaceful.

More recently we've added cell phone communications, smart-phones on our body, phone towers on telephone poles, and office buildings. We are being bombarded with EMF and EMR. Just as a negative co-worker can create psychic stress, these communication technologies can create EMF/EMR stress.

Here are a few tips to manage and mitigate this form of stress:

- Turn your cell phone to airplane mode as often as possible when the device is on your person.
- Turn it off completely when you can.
- Turn your Wi-Fi off when you sleep.
- Turn your breakers off if you can (leaving the refrigerator and any other critical appliances running).
- Use an earpiece and/or limit your conversations to a few minutes at a time.
- Know that being connected to laptops, cellphones, or tablets while they are plugged in is far more detrimental as you are exposed to magnetic waves, which can cause inflammation in your body.

Inflammation is a key component of aging, and chronic inflam-mation simply breaks the body down and opens us up for disease. So, watch it!

One great way to help balance out all the electricity EMF/EMR is to spend time in nature. Being outside has its own frequency that will tune you up from a low level to a higher vibration. This can counter the effects of EMF/EMR exposure as well as energize your reserves. To take it to the next level, take your shoes off and ground your feet into the earth.

Chemical Stress

Since the dawn of the industrial revolution, we have been pumping billions of pounds of toxic compounds into the environment every year. We all know what it feels like to be in a densely populated congested polluted city. Do you feel like taking a shower and lying down after a long hot day in a dirty city? That's called stress relief!

Environmental degradation and the toxic burden are taking its toll on our health. Add to this the so-called "safe" levels of preservatives, food coloring, additives, flavorings, pharmaceutical drugs flushed into the municipal water supply, as well as PCB's, phthalates, dioxins, and neurotoxins, and it's easy to see how we are all subjected to chemical stress on a daily basis.

Buying organic food is probably the #1 way we can help mitigate this for our own tissues and biochemistry as well as for the world around us. Be cognizant of your environment and lower your exposure to toxic chemicals. It is a good idea to be vigilant about what you put in your mouth, what you put on your skin, what you spray in your yard, etc.

Clean your clothes and house with non-toxic, organic, and natural substances. The great thing is that there are so many options available to us of natural solutions that are far superior to their toxic counterparts.

2010

My wife was pregnant with our second child, and we had just moved into a beautiful penthouse apartment overlooking Santa Monica Bay. It was a hot, dry summer, and the 1,800-square-foot apartment sparkled in the afternoon sun. The walls were freshly painted, and the carpets were new. We were in heaven.

The last trimester of my wife's pregnancy was difficult. She was suffering from allergies and started to develop preeclampsia. Her blood pressure became dangerously high, and her OB/GYN was worried about hypertension. On December 10, 2010, the doctors induced labor, and our beautiful baby daughter Athena was born three weeks early.

My mother-in-law came to help. As Christmas approached, the Southern California evenings started to dip down into the 40s. We turned the furnace on for the first time, and soon everyone was sick. Upper respiratory infections lingered for weeks and months at a time. Our energy was sapped. We felt lethargic. Our brains were in a deep fog.

I ignored the signs. I thought it was just a factor of being a new dad. I was solidly into my 40s and figured I was just paying the price for procreating at this later stage of my life.

I was also stressed financially. In 2012, one of my primary businesses went into a tailspin. I had a couple of partners, and many of the factors were beyond my control. Times were hard. My wife volunteered to go back to work in the fashion industry. She still had some contacts and could keep the lights on and food on our table. I volunteered to take over her duties at home. We were doing the best we could under the circumstances, but our lives were wildly out of balance.

If you never raised two young children, you have no idea how to prepare. You really don't know what you don't know. I thought I could step in and easily take over for my wife. I was sorely mistaken. If this was a romantic comedy, this would be the part where I hand my wife her lunch, give her a kiss, and tell her not to worry about a thing. Then everything would go comically awry in a music montage. The baby would cry all day for her mother, no matter what I did to amuse her. Her older brother, unsupervised, would paint the walls, overflow the toilet, and pee in the refrigerator. Slowly but surely, my optimistic demeanor would be replaced with anger, then quiet resignation. My wife would have to work late, and dinner would get burned and go uneaten. I'd fail miserably at the nighttime rituals and the three of us would each end the sequence crying alone in our beds, waiting for mom to come home.

Unfortunately, this was no romantic comedy. My wife was exhausted. I was beyond stressed. We were coughing and wheezing all the time. Then our son, Little Troy, got pneumonia. He woke up crying and coughing, and we could tell right away something was wrong. We went to the emergency room, and they admitted him on the spot. He spent three nights in the hospital, and those bills just piled on top of the unbearable strain we were already under.

This wasn't normal. How does a healthy 7-year-old kid get pneumonia in Santa Monica? Why can't my wife even go into the second bedroom without violent coughing spasms?

I started asking around and learned from my neighbors that several years before, the sprinkler system in our apartment had broken on more than one occasion. Alberto, the old guy who lived downstairs, told me he had seen water standing ankle-deep in our apartment. WTF?!

Everything started to click into place. Eleanor was this firecracker of an old lady who lived three doors down. She was always going in and out of the hospital, and we would take care of her plants. I had noticed water stains everywhere in her apartment but thought she must have had some kind of plumbing issue. Now I was beginning to fear the worst.

We had our place tested and, sure enough, they discovered Stachybotrys, Aspergillus, and Penicillium molds. Stachybotrys, or black mold, is the most dangerous. The spores produce mycotoxins that can be extremely harmful if inhaled, eaten, or even touched.

And we'd been living there for two years!

I took the kids camping for three weeks to try to heal them in nature while my wife looked for another apartment. Unfortunately for us, Silicon Beach was heating up. Snapchat and Tinder had taken off, and rents in Santa Monica were skyrocketing. It was easily going to cost us $1,000 more per month to rent another place.

New kid. New job. New house. The "Big Three" classic stressors of modern life, and we were living a trifecta. A perfect storm of stress.

The move almost killed us. We spent our entire savings, and the bills were piling up. The fabric of our marriage started to fray. There were fights about money. There were disagreements about parenting styles. Insults and long silences. It was a total shit show.

That's when I started having thoughts of suicide. I was in a very dark place. I would lie awake at night, listening to my gut gurgling. My digestion was shot. I was constipated and hadn't taken a shit in a week. Was this rock bottom? Unfortunately, not yet.

I turned to the one person in the world who influenced me the most, who helped me recover from my mental, physical, and emotional wounds: Paul Chek.

Paul's teachings have shaped my understanding and mastery of the 9 Pillars, but since this is a chapter on movement, let me talk about three things, in particular, that helped me heal: Iyengar Yoga, Qigong, and Tai Chi.

Iyengar Yoga

I began my movement recovery with Iyengar Yoga. This form of Hatha yoga was developed by B.K.S. Iyengar and popularized in his bestselling 1966 book *Light on Yoga*. This gentle form of yoga focuses on precision of alignment in the different postures (asanas) along with breath control (pranayama).

There are over 200 asanas and 14 different types of pranayama, ranging from basic to advanced. Students work gradually, moving from simple to more complex poses to develop mind, body, and spirit in a step-by-step approach. Props, such as belts, blankets, and blocks, enable people young and old to perform the asanas correctly while minimizing the risk of injury.

Focusing on the structural alignment of the body helps unite mind, body, and spirit. Fewer, slower movements are prioritized over speed and number of reps. Strength, mobility, and balance are restored.

Qigong

In Chinese, qi (pronounced "chi") means "life force" and gong means "cultivation." Qigong is a holistic system of body posture, movement, breathing, and meditation techniques with roots in Chinese medicine, philosophy, and martial arts.

Qigong involves graceful, choreographed movements inspired by animals in nature, restoring balance to the body and mind. I learned to stand on one foot and tie my shoe in some of my Qigong training.

Tai Chi

With Tai Chi, I learned to bring power and strength into my movements. Focusing on the yin and yang, I explored the duality of how seemingly contrary forces are interrelated.

Two sides of the same coin. Savage and saint. Light and dark, literally and figuratively, working together. I let go of my anger. Darkness was not to be loathed or feared but accepted as a natural part of life. Once I accepted this in my mind, my body relaxed. I felt better in mind, body, and spirit.

Spoiler alert: this was a five-year process. From 2012 to 2017, my movements focused on walking, restorative yoga, Qigong, and Tai Chi. After five long years, I worked the mycotoxins out of my body and finally had all 9 Pillars in alignment. Only then did I go back to the gym and start lifting weights again. It was my 50th year, and I got ripped. But unfortunately, 2012 was not rock bottom. There was more darkness to come.

Movement is a form of medicine that helps to keep you mentally, physically, and emotionally healthy. Here are a few tips to help you build your Movement Pillar.

Assessment – Before you begin, do an honest assessment of where you are and where you want to go. Check the credentials of any trainer you work with and stay away from the hacks and meatheads who can do more harm than good. If you are a do-it-yourselfer, then do your homework first to avoid injury. I recommend starting with Paul Chek's *How to Eat, Move, and Be Healthy.*

Walking – Walking is the perfect expression of how the human body was meant to move through time and space. Walk barefoot in the grass or in nature as often as you can.

Iyengar Yoga – This gentle form of yoga focuses on precision of alignment in different postures (asanas) along with breath control (pranayama). Focusing on the structural alignment of the body helps unite mind, body, and spirit.

Qigong – This holistic system of body posture, movement, breathing, and meditation involves graceful choreographed movements inspired by animals in nature. It can help restore balance to body and mind.

Tai Chi – This ancient form of Chinese martial arts cultivates the life energy (qi) within and helps it flow smoothly and powerfully through the body. Tai Chi embraces duality – yin and yang – and helps you see the interconnectedness of seemingly contrary forces in yourself and the natural world.

In this chapter, I outlined the **7 Factors of Stress** and gave you some strategies for dealing with them. Here is a recap:

1. **Physical Stress** – Don't buy into the "no pain, no gain" myth. Let your body rest if it needs to.
2. **Digital Communications Stress** – We're in the midst of a grand technological experiment, and no one yet knows the full impact that it has on your health. Be mindful of how much digital communication you consume.

3. **Psychic Stress** – Surround yourself with people who don't rob you of your positive energy.

4. **Nutritional Stress** – #JERF (just eat real food).

5. **Thermal Stress** – Be prepared for temperature changes in natural and artificial environments. Have layers and hats available for different situations.

6. **Electromagnetic Fields (EMF) and Electromagnetic Radiation (EMR) Stress** – Turn off phones, Wi-Fi, and electricity when you can, and walk barefoot in the grass to ground yourself.

7. **Chemical Stress** – Eat organic food and eliminate toxic chemicals (such as cleaning and gardening supplies) from your home environment.

BREATH

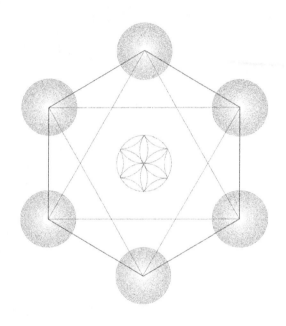

CHAPTER FIVE

"The mind is the king of the senses,
but the breath is the king of the mind."

Hatha Yoga Pradipika

2016

WE MOVED A few more times over the next couple of years, chased out by skyrocketing rents, always searching for that place we could truly call "home." Each move was more stressful than the last. Money was tight and we continued to fight. We said things we shouldn't have. Then we stopped saying things at all.

We began to avoid each other, which was hard in our 1,200-square-foot pad. But we managed. She took the bedroom. I slept on the couch. I got up early with the kids. When she finished her hour-long commute at the end of the day, I'd busy myself putting the kids to bed. If I was in the bedroom with Little Troy, she'd be in the bathroom with Athena. We passed each other like ghosts, never making eye contact.

We were both exhausted. There were dark shadows under her eyes, and her once-perfect posture crouched forward as if she'd aged 30 years. My breathing was faulty, my digestion shot. After the kids went to sleep, I'd slip out for a long walk along the beach to clear my head, and with any luck, she'd be asleep before I got back. In this way, we dammed up our emotions and let the stagnation set in.

It was a stressful time. I was riddled with anxiety. There is no doubt I was suffering from depression. Being in front of the camera, trying to be creative was hard enough without all the extra pressure. Something had to change.

I'd heard a motivational speaker say that your income is the average of the five dudes you hang out with the most, so I was open to expanding my network and adding some high-net-wealth individuals to my inner circle. I met Trevor, a successful producer who had his sights set on becoming a mogul, and we really hit it off. He was throwing a dinner party at his house in the Hollywood Hills, and he invited me to come.

I was 49 years old by this time, and my partying days were far behind me. But this was a good opportunity to network, and I might have some fun. It had been a long time since I'd had a boy's night out. I was just going to have dinner and head home early. I had a ton of work to do, and I didn't want to be exhausted the next day.

One of Trevor's oldest buddies, Dmitri, had just come back from a golfing trip in Scotland. He was a big single malt guy and had splurged on some thousand-dollar-a-bottle Macallan. In fact, he bought a case of it. We were celebrating Trevor's latest success, and Dmitri brought out a bottle to toast.

"I'm good," I said as he passed shot glasses around to the six of us at the table.

"C'mon, Troy," Dmitri grinned. "It's not every day you're offered the nectar of the gods!"

Everyone else at the table agreed and raised their glasses. I grabbed mine. I'd just have one. And so it goes.

I finally left the party at 1:15 am and headed south on Western. I figured traffic on Santa Monica Freeway would be reasonable at this time of the morning, and I might still be able to get six hours of sleep before I had to get up and make breakfast for the kids.

That's when the flashing blue lights caught my eye. Fuck! The cop said I was going 50 in a 35. I apologized. He asked me if I'd been drinking. I lied.

"Just one, but that was hours ago." "Uh huh. Step out of the car please."

DUI

Uri and I hadn't really spoken in weeks, so when I called at 3:00 am and told her that I needed to be bailed out of jail, things went from bad to worse.

The black mold had taken a serious toll on us. The moves and the financial stress put us in a pressure cooker. Being parents of two young children left us exhausted, and the DUI was the final straw.

"We can't afford this, Troy," Uri told me. "This will ruin us." I was afraid she might be right.

The fabric of our marriage was irreparably damaged, and before long, the inevitable came.

"I want a divorce."

It was like getting coldcocked. I gasped for breath. I didn't want a divorce. I loved my wife. I loved my family. We were going through a rough patch, but doesn't every couple? And from a practical standpoint, I really couldn't afford it. We were barely getting by under one roof. How would we pay for two? And what about the kids? Would we have joint custody? Would I have to get approval from the court to see my own children? How had everything turned so thoroughly to shit?

We tried counseling. We tried working through our issues. We tried talking. We tried silence. Nothing worked. One night after the kids went to bed, we both looked at each other and knew the time had come.

"Okay," I said. "You win. You can have your divorce."

She didn't say anything. I couldn't tell if she was hurt or relieved. She just looked at me for a long time, then turned and left the room. I could hear the bedroom door close at the end of the hall.

I sank down onto the couch and cried.

I woke at 4:00 am drenched in sweat. My heart was beating fast. I was falling in my dream and lurched awake with a sense of vertigo. My stomach was churning, and I thought I might puke.

It took me a few seconds to recognize my own living room. And then like an aftershock, it all came flooding back to me.

"You can have your divorce."

You can survive three weeks without food, three days without water, and three minutes without oxygen.

Oxygen is vital for life, and I was literally gasping for air.

If this wasn't a panic attack, it was doing a pretty good imitation. I felt disconnected from my body. I was adrift in a psychic sewer of anger and humiliation. Lost. Drowning.

Alone. I was reaching out desperately for a lifeline. And so my soul cashed in some chips.

My spiritual journey has taught me many things. I believe in soul contracts; the concept that we make agreements with other souls before we are born, and that these souls will come into our lives at certain times to teach us who we are, and who we are destined to be.

The next day, I was running a workshop in Venice, and who should walk through the door but Erik Casano (also known as Dr. Pee Pee Shivambu). We'd been following each other on social media for a little while, but I'd never met him before. Erik was a fascinating character who had been on his own spiritual journey. He was a Swedish national living in the U.S. who developed testicular cancer. Because Sweden has socialized medicine, he went back there for treatment. After the first round of chemo, the doctors told him they wanted to remove his lymph nodes.

"Um...I think I need my lymph nodes," he said.

He decided to take a different path. He researched ancient and alternative medical practices, traveled with Sherpas high in the Himalayas, and learned from mystic masters. In the end, he landed on Shivambu (urine therapy) as a cure. Two years later, when he went back to the hospital in Sweden, the doctors were amazed.

Erik should have been dead, but instead he was cancer-free. How had this been achieved?

"I drank my own pee," he said with a gleam in his eye. They didn't want to hear any more.

Erik had also spent years studying breath work and had seen the transformative effect it had on his life. Our soul contract led him to me at the moment in my life that I needed him most.

He had picked up on my faulty breathing in the morning session. He could feel the tension in my body and sense the anxiety in my mind. He could see the exhaustion in my face.

At our first break, he came up to me and said, "Do you mind if I teach you some breath work? It'll only take five minutes, and I think it will really help you."

"Sure," I said. I am always open to learning something new.

As we got down on our knees, he said, "This is emergency breath work. If you don't do any other breath work during the day, just do this one."

"Take a yoga block and prop your butt up," he instructed, doing the same. "Some people do this sitting cross-legged, but I find the spine drops a little in that position. This allows your diaphragm to poke open a little."

"Now put your hands on your knees. We're going to breathe in and out through the nose intensely. On the 11th breath, hold it as long as you can."

And so we did. After a minute, he relaxed his shoulders and exhaled slowly.

"Do it again, but this time, hold it on the 16th breath." We repeated the cycle, dropping our shoulders and exhaling at the end.

"Last one. This is the kicker!" he smiled. "Hold it this time on the 21st breath. But instead of relaxing and exhaling slowly, squeeze your perineum – you know, that diamond-shaped area between your genitals and your anus. This will pump the energy up your spine into your pineal gland."

Nineteen. Twenty. Twenty-one. Hold it. Squeeze.

I felt my qi, my prana, my life force ripple through me. I felt the vibration move up my spine. Oxygen filled my brain. Dopamine and serotonin flooded my system. As I settled down on the yoga block and let my shoulders drop, a smile filled my face.

Dr. Pee Pee Shivambu grinned like a kid who'd just shown his little brother an amazing new trick.

"You're going to sleep better tonight," he promised. And you know what? I did.

Don't get me wrong. I still had anxiety. I still had depression. One breath work session was not a cure. My marriage was still falling apart. Try as we might, we could not work through the emotional stagnation that filled the space between us. The divorce marched forward. Papers were signed, and arrangements were made. Like many parents going through a divorce, we worried about the impact our separation would have on the kids. We wanted them to feel safe. Secure. Loved. And unlike so many others I'd seen, we didn't wage war on each other.

I didn't want to hurt her. She didn't want to hurt me. No acrimony. No victims. She didn't rub my nose in the DUI, which ended up costing more than $15k and stretched our already-tight finances to the breaking point.

There were many nights I woke up on the couch or curled up on a mattress after she moved out, gasping for air. My gut boiled and gurgled all night long. I had dark thoughts. More than once, I thought about ending it all. I was in a nightmare, and I didn't know how to wake myself up.

But I kept breathing. Oxygen kept me alive, minute by minute, day by day. Erik started coming over to my house and teaching me other techniques.

"This one's called the Bhastrika," he said as we crossed our legs on the living room floor. "It's a traditional yoga breathing exercise to help increase your life force or prana."

"Bhastrika is used to energize the body and clarify the mind. It's a powerful technique, so you need to go easy."

He'd gotten to know me pretty well and had seen how aggressive I could be.

"This one can make you a bit light-headed. I wouldn't want you to crack your skull," he smiled.

"Sit up tall," he said. "Relax your shoulders. Take a deep breath in through your nose." "Now let it out."

"Now, breathe forcefully through your nose, like a bellows. In and out. One per second. Ten sharp breaths in. Ten sharp breaths out."

"Out from the diaphragm. Don't be a neck breather," he smiled, knowing my faulty breathing. "Belly moves, in and out. Head, neck, shoulders still."

He counted off a 15-second break, and then we did a set of 20. We took a 30-second break, and then did 30 more breaths. I was getting a little lightheaded, but not dizzy. I could feel the dopamine and serotonin coursing through my veins.

"One more?" he asked, checking if I was okay.

I smiled and nodded. We did another 30-breath set. 90 breaths in all. Sharp bellows in and out.

The sharp breaths activated the sympathetic nervous system, then the parasympathetic nervous system kicked in, and a wave of calm passed over me.

Wow!

Another time, Erik took me through my first Holotropic

Breathwork® exercise. Pioneered by Stanislav Grof in the 1960s, this technique was meant to simulate some of the same conscious-altering experiences that his earlier LSD therapy had explored. After LSD was criminalized following the Timothy Leary era at Harvard, Dr. Grof created this technique to access non-ordinary states of consciousness without the use of the LSD molecule.

From the Greek "holos," meaning "whole," and "trepein," meaning "moving in the direction of," Holotropic breathing is an intense approach to self-exploration. The purpose is to move you toward your whole self or wholeness.

Working in pairs (Sitters and Breathers) in a ritualistic setting with evocative music, Holotropic Breathwork® is designed to open up different states of consciousness.

Breathers lie on a mat with eyes closed and do aggressive breathing that creates a hyperventilated state. The sitter is merely present to assist, not to interfere or guide the experience.

An hour into it, I found myself curled up in a fetal position, experiencing a "rebirth." I was aware of being conceived, of growing in my mother's womb, of passing through the birth canal, of taking my first breath.

Similar to my work in the Amazon with ayahuasca, this technique gave me a completely different perspective on my life. The anxiety and fears that haunted my waking life, now seemed so insignificant. What I had thought were enormous and undefeatable challenges were mere trifles. Seen from a certain angle, the shadows these things cast were terrifying, but to view them now, I wondered how I could ever have been frightened of something so inconsequential.

We are the all-powerful, self-healing children of God. We are endowed with unimaginable grace and love. Life is beautiful.

My pillars were in disarray. Stress was upending my sleep, my digestion, my immune system, my thoughts and emotions. Breath work gave me a powerful tool to stand the pillars on end again. Oxygen, that most vital element, could be channeled. Its powers harnessed. Its life-giving force multiplied.

You see, at a cellular level, our bodies need oxygen to survive. I won't bore you with a long explanation of cellular respiration, but it is essential in turning glucose into energy that our bodies can use.

RippedAt50 is, above all things, a book about health optimization. I want to be as healthy as I can be. I want to live a long and happy life, free from pain and disease. My body has been engineered to sustain life at an optimum level, but stressors can inhibit this efficiency. By understanding how all of these things are interconnected, I hoped to optimize my health, achieve my dreams, and leave a meaningful legacy behind.

Cellular respiration is a fundamental building block underlying everything. It is the set of metabolic processes and reactions that converts biochemical energy from nutrients into adenosine triphosphate (ATP). Carbon dioxide is a waste product, and cellular respiration moves that out of your body.

In humans, this cellular respiration is aerobic, which means that cells need oxygen to create ATP. In an optimum system, the cells get all the oxygen they need to produce the ATP to power your body. Suboptimal systems can starve the cells of the oxygen they need, forcing them to turn to less optimal ways to create ATP, such as fermentation, which creates lactic acid.

In simple terms, it is easy to see how respiration affects cellular respiration.

On a macro level, the gas exchange between plants and animals is a fundamental cycle of life. Animals need oxygen to survive and produce carbon dioxide as a waste product.

Plants need carbon dioxide for their own cellular respiration (photosynthesis) and produce oxygen as a waste product. Mother Nature has built a beautiful, symbiotic system that has sustained life on earth for millions of years.

My spiritual journey has taught me not only how interrelated the different systems of my body are to each other, but also how my body is connected to the earth. Clean water, clean soil, and clean air are the birthright of every human on earth. We cannot separate our own health from the health of the earth any more than we can separate our digestion from our sleep.

Consider the fact that an acre of trees produces enough oxygen for about 18 people to live for a year. That same acre of trees also absorbs enough carbon dioxide to offset a car driven 26,000 miles. More than 20% of all the oxygen on earth is produced in the Amazon rain forests.

Now consider the fact that we're losing about 1.5 acres of rain forest every second. In the time it took you to read that sentence, the earth lost enough trees to keep more than 100 people alive for a year. How long is this sustainable? When will we pass a point of no return? How long can the earth sustain human life at its present scale?

It is enough to take your breath away.

Living a life of optimal health means that I must also think about the health of the planet I live on. I was determined to speak my dream into existence.

I am a humble, kind, and gentle man. My mission is to raise human consciousness and change all systems. My vision is clean air, water, soil, and equitable systems for all mankind... in my lifetime.

These breathing exercises were instrumental to my healing process. One important part of my soul contract had been fulfilled. I was learning who I was and who I was destined to be.

As we went through our divorce, breathing became my lifeline. Every morning I would lie flat, breathing in through my nose and out through my mouth. Big deep breaths. I let two-thirds of the air fill my stomach and the last one-third fill my lungs. 90 deep breaths oxygenated my body and cleared my mind. It got me up to feed my kids and helped me have a normal day. Or at least as "normal" a day as I could have as my marriage fell apart around me.

Because of the DUI, I wasn't driving, and my sole method of transportation was my mountain bike. As my breathing got more intentional, I focused on getting air into my pelvic floor. I'd learned enough anatomy and physiology to begin to understand the connection between the diaphragm, the transverse abdominis, and the pelvic floor.

I never could have gotten my six-pack abs without these breathing exercises. The abs were always there – I just had to let them come out. All the dieting and fasting, along with all the crunches in the world, could not have done it alone. For years I had been flexing my stomach muscles to look good in front of the camera, but this had created a tension in my diaphragm that was prohibiting it from working as it should have. Breath work helped me reprogram my physiology through breathing to get *RippedAt50*.

There was some psychology I had to unravel. There were movements that brought my musculoskeletal and nervous systems back into balance. I was on a psycho-spiritual journey, delving deep into my own consciousness. I had to be mindful of every aspect, to assess and repair the systems that were not optimal, and then move them from my waking life to my unconscious life. Now I don't have to think about my breathing as much. It is a natural, automatic process. Optimized.

Paul Chek played no small part in my breathing education. One of the Tai Chi movements he taught me was breathing squats. Standing on one leg, you bring your arms up over your head like the wings of a stork as you breathe in deeply. Then, you slowly put your arms down and squat as you exhale. At the same time, you bring the other leg up, squeezing all the gasses out of your body. Another similar movement was the Stork Walk. This helped me reprogram my breathing apparatus. The diaphragm and the rib cage open up.

I learned about hard breathing. I learned about retention breathing – with retention on both the inhale and the exhale.

As I write this now, at age 53, I basically have a gorilla body. I've worked very hard at optimizing each system, at perfecting each of the 9 Pillars. My digestion is better. I am pooping better. I am not carrying any extra fat. I am breathing optimally. I've worked on my body mechanics, my posterior chain, so that my posture is functionally fit. My nutrition is on point. I sleep well. My thoughts are healthy. My relationships are deep and fulfilling. I get into nature and walk barefoot in the grass. I live my dream.

This midlife crisis was the perfect storm. It could have destroyed me, but instead it forced me to put everything together. I could never be what I am now without these experiences. I am grateful for them. All of them. No victims.

Breathing saw me through.

You can survive three weeks without food, three days without water, and three minutes without oxygen. Breath work can help you channel this most vital of elements to fuel your body and relax your mind. Here are a few simple exercises to help you build your Breath Pillar.

5-Minute Daily Breath Work Exercise

If you do only one breathing exercise, do this one. I like to do this one first thing in the morning to pump oxygen into my brain and body and regulate my sleep patterns.

- Get down on your knees.
- Use a yoga block or pillow to prop up your butt and open up your diaphragm.
- Sit up straight and put your hands on your knees.
- Breathe in and out intensely through your nose.

    o On the **11th breath**, hold it for as long as you can.

    ▪ Relax, drop your shoulders, and exhale slowly.

    o Repeat, but this time hold on the **16th breath.**

    ▪ Relax, drop your shoulders, and exhale slowly.

    o Repeat, but this time hold on the **21st breath.**

    ▪ **Don't exhale yet!**

    ▪ Squeeze your perineum – the area between your genitals and anus.

    ▪ Feel the energy pump up your spine and into your pineal gland.

Bhastrika

The name of this traditional yoga breathing exercise means "bellows." It can be a little intense, so take it easy when first trying it so that you don't get dizzy and hit your head.

- Sit cross-legged.
- Relax your shoulders.
- Breathe forcefully (like a bellows) through your nose, once per second.

  o Remember to use your diaphragm instead of your chest. Your belly should move in and out when breathing.

  o Keep your head, neck, and shoulders still.

- Take 10 sharp breaths followed by a 15-second break.
- Take 20 sharp breaths followed by a 30-second break.
- Take 30 sharp breaths followed by a 30-second break.
- Take 30 sharp breaths.
- Relax.

This 90-breath exercise activates both your sympathetic and parasympathetic nervous systems, producing clarity and calm.

THOUGHT

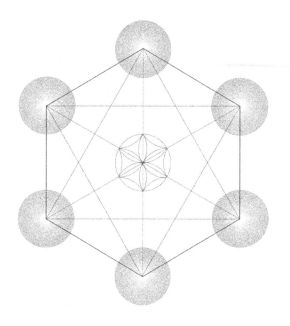

CHAPTER SIX

*"Whatever the mind can conceive and believe,
it can achieve."*

Napoleon Hill

2017

MY DIVORCE WAS final. Uri and I lived in separate apartments about a mile away, and we split custody. I finally hit rock bottom and I was now on my way back up. The anxiety wasn't completely gone, but it was subsiding. I often slept the entire night without waking up in a panic. I was healing.

My brother Shawn was in town with his son for a bodybuilding competition, and he actually called me this time. Sometimes I wouldn't even hear from him when he came into town, but this time was different. Uri and I met them for breakfast (despite our divorce we were still deeply connected, in many ways we were still family) and while having her there eased the tension I was expecting, the exchange between my brother and I was still as awkward as I expected.

Shawn and I never really got along. Maybe he thought I stole his thunder. He was only 1½ years old when I came along, so he didn't get to be the baby for long. After my stepfather was arrested, the family fell apart, and we were separated for many years.

When we finally reunited in our 20s, I had a dream that we would bond like brothers should, that we would confide in each other, have each other's backs. If not best friends, then at least good brothers. But that never happened either.

We were both pretty opinionated and both pretty aggressive. When we disagreed, things got heated. And we disagreed on a lot of things. So I had a brother in the world, but we were really strangers. And by extension, his family and mine were somewhat estranged.

Shawn had fought his own demons. He had been hooked on heroin and almost died from an overdose. Back in 1991, when Shawn was trying to clean up his own life, Tony Robbins had just released *Awaken the Giant Within*. Shawn bought all the cassette tapes and would listen to them over and over again. They worked. Shawn got through his addictions and became enormously successful in the fitness world.

I was just rebounding from the lowest point in my life. My marriage had disintegrated. I had gotten a DUI and didn't even have a driver's license. My financial status was precarious. Maybe I was jealous, or self-conscious, or both. At any rate, I was relieved when breakfast was over. There were no fights. No angry words were spoken. No acrimony or recriminations. We caught up. We were nice to each other. We hugged at the end like real brothers should. If you were watching from across the street, you might even think we had a loving relationship.

On the drive home, Uri said, "I invited them to dinner. 6:00." "What?" I gasped. "Why would you do that?"

"He's your brother, Troy. You need to open your heart to him." "I've tried. He's not interested."

"You should try again."

I knew that was true, but my stomach squirmed at the thought of it.

"We'll end up having a fight," I said. "We always do. We have different opinions on just about everything."

"Don't fight with him then. Just listen."

Just because he was 18 months older than me, I was supposed to *listen* to him? To *him*?

"He's just such an asshole," I said finally. It wasn't a good argument. I just had to get it off my chest.

"Maybe you're the asshole," she said as we pulled up in front of my apartment. She looked me in the eyes, waiting for the smartass comeback she had grown to hate.

Maybe I surprised her this time. I shrugged my shoulders, smiled, and said, "Maybe you're right."

I got out and started toward the door.

"Be there at 4. And bring the food. You're cooking."

She drove off, and I went inside and did some breath work. Maybe I *was* the asshole. But people can change.

Cooking for my brother and nephew could be challenging. Being so into fitness, they're pretty opinionated about their diets. We'd had our food spats in the past, but dinner actually turned out pretty great. The kids loved playing with their older cousin, and he was great to them. They laughed all night, and it made my heart sing to see them so happy.

Uri cleaned up, then took the kids for a walk on the beach while Shawn and I caught up.

We didn't have many "old times" to catch up on, but we managed to reminisce about the old house in Connecticut near the lake.

"Remember that treehouse we built beside the lake?" Shawn asked.

"Sure. I especially remember you pushing me out of it," I joked. "You could have killed me!"

"But you landed on that inner tube, bounced up in the air, landed on your feet and said 'I'm gonna kill you, Shawn!'" he squeaked in a high voice, trying to impersonate the five-year-old me.

We both laughed. There were a few fond memories of our youth still intact. "Remember that black dog we'd have to walk past to get there?"

"Sparky," I remembered. "That dog used to terrify me." "Remember the day he stopped terrifying you?"

No. I had no memory of that at all.

"That's the day we broke the saw," Shawn said.

"I remember that," I said, thinking back to that day. It must have been 1970 or 1971. I must have been five or six. Funny to think how it was no problem for us to use all the power tools in the garage back then. "We were making wooden swords, but then you wanted to see if that old band saw could cut a metal pipe."

"Yeah," my brother laughed. "We took our swords and ran after that." "We played King of the Castle in the treehouse until it started to get dark." "But when it was time to go home, you refused."

"I did?" I asked. I didn't remember that.

"You said Sparky was going to try to bite you, so you weren't going home," he said. "I figured you were really afraid of the beating we'd get for breaking the saw."

"Yeah, *you* broke the saw, but we both got a beating."

"Yeah, sorry about that," he said. "Anyway, I told you I'd teach you a trick. If you say 'I am not afraid of Sparky'..."

"One hundred times, you won't be afraid of that dog anymore." The memory suddenly flashed back into my mind. How had I so completely forgotten it?

"So you sat there and said, 'I am not afraid of Sparky' one hundred times, and after that, you were never afraid of that dog again. I saw the change come over your face. If I close my eyes, I can still see you as you were that day. You believed you were scared, and so you were. And then you decided you weren't scared, and you weren't. I think about that day all the time."

"You do? We've never talked about it."

"I thought that was the day you started hating me. I broke the saw, you took a beating, and you never seemed to like me as much after that."

We had moved pretty soon after that. Things changed. My brother and I grew apart, and then were separated for years.

"I've never hated you," I said honestly.

"I know. But the point I'm making is that the power is all right up here," he said, tapping an index finger to his temple. "It's the biggest lesson I've learned in life, that our *thoughts* create our reality. And I know this in my heart to be true because I witnessed you do it when you were five."

It was nice, not fighting with him for once.

Then he laid his hand on my arm and said, "Troy, I want to challenge you to do something. Will you accept?"

"Yes," I answered without a pause. If he was surprised, he didn't show it. "Do you know what a gratitude journal is?"

Isn't that self-explanatory? This is usually where our conversations would start to go off the rails. But I bit my lip.

"I've never done one," I said honestly.

"I want you to start. Tonight, before you go to sleep, I want you to write down three things you are grateful for. And tomorrow morning, when you wake up, I want you to write down three more things. I want you to do that for 100 days."

He slid a leather-bound journal across the table. "I'll write down five," I said. Challenge accepted.

We spent the next few hours in the first real conversation we'd had in decades. Years ago, he had gone through his own crisis. His thoughts had been dark. Self-destructive. Heroin had nearly killed him.

"The gratitude journal changed my life," he told me. "I used to be so angry Troy, you have no idea."

"I think I've got a pretty good idea," I laughed.

"Yeah, I bet you do. Which is why I think this will work for you too. I used to only focus on the negative. What I *didn't* have. What I *couldn't* achieve. And I put myself in a prison. A prison of my own mind.

"Then I started writing things down, and everything changed. Nothing in life has any meaning, except the meaning we give it. We literally create the world we live in. Not figuratively. Literally. If you believe that you'll fail, you will fail. But if you believe you will succeed, then anything is possible. It all starts with a positive mental attitude. And gratitude, brother, is the perfect antidote for darkness."

I leaned forward. He had my attention. "How do you mean?" I asked. "Have you heard of dark matter?" he asked.

"Sure," I said. "Scientists did all these gravitational calculations on galaxies and can't explain why they're doing what they're doing. For our understanding of gravity to work, there must be matter they can't see, so they call it dark matter."

"That's right," he nodded, seeming impressed. "Not all male models are idiots," I smiled.

"They say dark matter makes up 85% of the universe. Scientists can observe the gravitational effects, but they can't fully explain why the universe works the way it does. I can't show you a diagram to explain why gratitude works. I can't show you the gratitude molecule under a microscope, but that doesn't mean it doesn't exist. I can observe the effects it has. I can measure and quantify them. I see it every day."

Shawn was getting excited now. He had the same look on his face as when we were kids.

"You can't have gratitude without love. And love..." he paused, trying to find just the right words, "love changes the chemistry of the brain, reverses the polarity of our dark thoughts. Turns them from dark to light. Love connects our thoughts to God, to the Almighty, to the universe.

"I was in a low place. I didn't love myself. I tried pretty hard to destroy myself," he continued. "The gratitude journal made me realize how blessed I was. How loved I was. And with that frame of mind, I started to love myself."

"The way I see it, you've got so much to be grateful for. You've got two beautiful children. You live in Santa Monica and go to the beach every day. From what I can tell, you don't have a real job. You do *what* you want, *when* you want. You work with who you want. You eat organic foods. You're in the best shape I think I've ever seen you.

You're tan. You've got six-pack abs in your 50s. Most people on the planet would trade places with you in a heartbeat. Some of the most successful guys I know would pay a fortune to have what you've got. Your mind is sharp. You've got loving relationships. You've got the world by the tail, and you don't even know it.

"And here's one thing I'm grateful for," he said, looking me right in the eyes. "I'm grateful for you, Troy. I'm glad you're my little brother, and I love you."

"I'm grateful for you too, Shawn," I confessed. That night, I wrote down five things:

1. I am grateful for my brother, Shawn. He challenged me to start this gratitude journal.
2. I am grateful for Uri. She always calls out my bullshit.
3. I am grateful for my son, Little Troy. He reminds me of Jesse.
4. I am grateful for my daughter, Athena. She shows me every day what unconditional love looks like.
5. I am grateful for my mother, Ann. She gave me this wonderful life I live.

The universe is a mysterious place. Studies show that plants will grow more if you talk nicely to them. Water will freeze in different crystalline structures depending on the words you speak to them at the moment of freezing. Gratitude attracts. Providence will rise up to meet you and bring you the things you are thankful for.

The next morning, I wrote down five more things. I did this religiously for six months, pouring my heart out onto paper. I never realized how many blessings I had. I eventually began to realize I was thankful for some "bad" things too.

> Day 34: I am grateful for the DUI. It made me realize, once and for all, that alcohol is bad for me.

I felt the change in me. Being thankful changed my state of mind. The anxiety melted away. So did my fear of failure. My fear of financial disaster. All fear is really just a fear of death in the end. Those fears began to evaporate.

I was so blessed. I was endowed with a mind, a heart, and a soul. I had a nose to smell with. Eyes to see with. Ears to hear with. Fingers to touch with. The prison of my mind was imaginary, and the key to escape was in my hand the whole time. I just needed to use it.

> Day 73: I am grateful for the love I experience daily from my friends and family. It shows me that I am loved, even when I have a hard time loving myself.

My brother was right; gratitude was a great place to start. My thoughts were more positive, and I was happier.

Shawn and I didn't stay in touch. We returned to being strangers, but I hope someday we can reconnect and stay close. But the gratitude journal he challenged me to start was the beginning of a yet another transformation.

My spiritual journey led me into an exploration of thoughts, and as always, I plunged in with gusto. Just as I had reprogrammed my breathing and brought my body into balance with intention, I set about reprogramming my mindset.

When I thought of all the things that brought stress into my life, finances were always at or near the top of the list. If I had to guess, I'd say 75% of all the fights I'd had with my wife were about money. I'd grown up poor and had known financial instability my whole life. When I explored my own thoughts, I found that deep down, I really *expected* to be financially insecure. Of course, consciously, I've always wanted to succeed, to provide for my family, to enjoy a luxurious lifestyle. But peel away the layers, look a little deeper at my own thoughts, and I saw a different picture.

My mom used to joke that we were just unlucky. Bad things seemed to follow the Casey family around. She didn't even say it to complain, and she didn't even seem angry about it. Whenever something bad would happen, she'd say, "There's that old Casey Luck again." I just shrugged it off like a harmless joke. It was just a thing she said. After a while, I started saying it too.

Now I realized that this was not a harmless saying. This was far more damaging. If you repeat a thought often enough, you will begin to believe it. My explorations made me see that unconsciously, I had "Casey Luck." I *expected* bad things to happen, and so bad things happened. I expected money troubles, and those came too.

The good news is we have free will. My thoughts are my own, and I am free to think whatever I want! The bad news is that thoughts and habits can etch deep grooves in our psyches, and sometimes we have to take our medicine to escape from these negative pathways. Medicine can come in many forms. One form I don't particularly like – but which I know is good for me – is cold showers.

I don't like rolling out of a warm bed into a cold shower any more than you do. But I've seen the benefit this ritual makes on my mental health and since 2011, I have made it part of my daily ritual.

Too much in modern life is yang. We are inflamed by stressors in our bodies and in our minds. Cold water is a natural remedy. It is the yin water that helps balance us.

For most of our existence, Homo sapiens have bathed in natural water that was much colder than is common today. And in that respect, I think we've lost something vital Cold water is bracing. Uncomfortable even. But for me, cold water is invigorating.

I still began each morning with breath work. I would lie flat, breathing in through my nose and out through my mouth. Big deep breaths. Two-thirds of the air into the stomach, one-third into the lungs. My gut was getting better, but still not 100%. With me, it's always about the gut. I had worked with a Taoist practitioner who taught me some techniques that helped. So, while I breathed in the morning, I would massage one spot right under my rib cage and another toward the belly button that were just as hard as rocks. I suspected these were parts of the vagus nerve. The brain ganglia can get intertwined with the musculature and create stagnation in the 2nd and 3rd chakras.

Thoughts, like muscles, need to be exercised. Repetition builds neural pathways, reinforces ideas, and makes them grow.

I am a humble, kind, and gentle man.

This was my personal statement. This is what I aspired to be. If I repeated this thought to myself enough, I would come to believe it. And when I believe it is true, it will be so.

I am a humble, kind, and gentle man.

After my breath work, I would take a cold shower. Here is my basic routine:

I start with my extremities, letting the water splash over my arms and legs. Then I put my face into the water and feel the coldness spread from my forehead down my cheeks and around my neck. After 30 seconds or so I raise my arms and let the water run down each side of my body and then let the shower hit my chest for a long time. I just deal with it.

Finally, I raise my arms up over my head, turn, and let the cold water run from the crown of my head all the way down the spine.

I end with some breath of fire breathing, rapid and shallow. I shake myself off first, then towel dry.

And just like that, cold water has washed the slumber from my eyes and the drowsiness from my mind. I am sharp. Alert. Awake.

Cold showers douse the inflammation in my body and mind and give me focus. During this time of my life, cold showers have helped me reprogram my thinking.

I am a visual learner, so I've found vision boards to be one of the most effective ways to repeat an idea in my brain. I made one and hung it in my office as visual reinforcement for the mantra of myself. Humble was not just a word; it was my wife at prayer. Kind was a shoulder to cry on. Gentle was my brother Jesse. I would consciously stare at the vision board every day.

I am a humble, kind, and gentle man.

The images reinforced the thoughts; God only knows how many thousands of times my eyes scanned that text, recognized those images, and reinforced the thought of myself.

My mission is to raise human consciousness and change all systems.

Scott Peterson, my ayahuasca healer. The Shipibo women who taught young girls how to pull themselves out of poverty by making and selling tribal tapestries.

My vision is clean air, water, soil, and equitable systems for all mankind...in my lifetime.

Crystal clear streams, bright blue skies, rich black soil. I repeated the words over and over again. I said them out loud to myself. I focused on each picture. Burned the images into my memory, so that I could see them at night when I closed my eyes for sleep.

While cold showers are a daily dose of good medicine for me, sometimes I need something stronger. It was about this time in my life when I discovered ice baths.

When I was about 13, living by the lake in Connecticut, my brother fell through the ice one winter. The water was freezing, and at first I thought he would die. But he didn't. I think it actually made him stronger. Since then, I've waded in streams and rivers and I've swum in cold lakes.

But ice baths take that experience to the next level. It is strong medicine. I hate the taste of ayahuasca and have to mentally prepare myself every time I drink the plant medicine. But I know that it is good for me, so I take it. Likewise, I hate the sensation of putting my body in ice water. But I do it because I know that it is good for me.

Wim Hof, also known as "The Iceman," is a Dutch extreme athlete noted for his ability to withstand freezing temperatures. He has set Guinness World Records for swimming under ice and prolonged full-body contact with ice, and he still holds the record for a barefoot half-marathon on ice and snow. As Wim likes to say, "the cold is merciless, yet righteous." Submerging yourself in ice water is a death-defying act that can lead to purity.

Blood rushes from all extremities to the vital organs. Your sympathetic nervous system floods your body with chemicals to aid your survival. It activates ketogenesis and autogenesis. It balances your hormones and endocrine system. It strengthens your immune system and makes you more resilient and non-fragile. Everything non-essential is stripped away and your mind and body focus on one thing: survival.

By voluntarily putting yourself in this state, you can also test your spiritual foundation. The ice water allows you to let go of the trivial and forces you to focus on the essential. Martial arts masters try to prepare their students to deal with chaos. To adapt and survive, no matter what the battle may bring. In many ways, ice baths do the same thing.

But you can't think about it too much or you might talk yourself out of it. On the other side of it, once I've gotten out of the water and the feeling returns to my body, I always feel amazing. But the actual bath itself is something that takes courage and fortitude to attempt every single time.

In addition to the cold showers, I started doing ice baths two or three times a week and they pushed my thinking to a higher plane.

If you repeat a thought often enough, you will come to believe it. I was rewiring the circuitry of my brain, smoothing out the deep grooves left by older, destructive thoughts and slowly etching out new grooves for my thoughts to flow through. With each passing day, the new pathways grew deeper. The thoughts, which at first might have slipped off course at the slightest bump, now tracked solidly.

On top of the gratitude journal and vision boards, I added Binaural Beats to my sleep. This technique uses headphones to play tones of different frequencies in both ears. For instance, the right ear might get a tone at 240Hz, while the left ear gets a tone at 235Hz. The tones travel individually to your inferior colliculus where your brain perceives the dissonance between the two as a new 5Hz tone, and "tunes" to that new frequency.

Now, this tone is too low for you to hear, but it happens to be in the frequency of the brain waves during sleep. Thus, the theory goes, Binaural Beats can help with relaxation, reduce anxiety, increase creativity, and promote positive thinking.

Did they work? I thought and believed they did, so they did.

I wish I could isolate each piece of this experiment and measure the impact each factor had. Did the Binaural Beats reduce my anxiety more than the breath work? Did stimulating my vagus nerve have more impact than my nutrition? I can't give you a definitive answer. What I *can* say is that it was working. I felt better every day. My thoughts were clearer, and my emotions were more stable. My attitude was more positive.

And just like that, my life started to change. Opportunities that had eluded me in the past now came to me freely.

The mind is an embodied process. I am the sum total of all my thoughts, but I am the captain of those thoughts. Even if the wind was the same, I could use my sails to turn in a different direction.

I can't say that miracles happen overnight. They don't. By one measure, it took me more than 50 years to get here. But when I decided to change my thoughts, my body and my life changed with them.

I am living a miracle now. Every day is blessed. I don't do a gratitude journal now – I don't have to. I am just so grateful for everything, and so filled with love.

Building Your Thought Pillar

If you repeat a thought often enough to yourself, you will begin to believe it. And once you begin to believe it, it will become true. This is one of the great truths of life, hiding right in plain sight. We *literally* create our own reality. Here are some tips to help you build your Thought Pillar.

Gratitude Journal

Some clients have told me they don't need to do a gratitude journal because they are already grateful. I remind them that is like saying, "I don't need to eat organic because I already know that it is good for me." The mind is an embodied process, and positive change requires you to move beyond the theoretical and into the actual. Just as movement builds your body, thinking builds your mind. Daily exercise of both mind and body is important.

I would like to personally challenge you to do a gratitude journal for 100 days. Here's how:

- **Morning** – Every morning when you wake up, write down three things you are grateful for.
- **Night** – Every night before you go to sleep, write down three more things you are grateful for.
- **Extra Credit** – Embrace the duality of existence by finding light in the darkness.

Can you find gratitude in your worst and most painful experiences?

Doing this thought exercise for 100 days changed my life, and I think it can change yours too.

Personal Mission/Vision Statement

Remember the personal mission/vision statement we worked on to help you build your Legacy Pillar? The Thought Pillar can help you make that mission and vision a reality. Read it out loud to yourself. Commit it to memory. Think it over and over and over to yourself until

119

it becomes a part of you. Rewire your brain to believe that this personal mission/vision statement is true, and you will start to make it so.

Vision Boards

Seeing is believing. If you want to achieve something, creating a vision board can help you turn that dream into reality. Take your personal mission/vision statement and find the pictures that best represent it. Clip out the pictures and create a collage. You can use text in your design to reinforce key ideas. Hang it up in space where you'll see it often every day. Look at it as you recite your mission/vision statement to yourself.

Cold Showers

Rolling out of a warm bed into a cold shower is a healthy way to start the day. Start with your extremities, letting the water splash on your arms and legs, then put your face into the water. Get both sides of your torso, then let the water pound your chest and get your heart pumping. Just deal with it! Finish by letting the cold water run from the crown of your head down your spine. This daily dose of medicine helps wipe the sleep from your eyes and invigorate your mind for the day.

Ice Baths

The cold is merciless, but righteous! Don't think about it too much before you submerge your body in ice water for 1 – 3 minutes. This death-defying act forces the blood to rush to your vital organs, to fight for your very survival. It helps balance your hormones, strengthen your immune system, and test your spiritual foundation. Learn to be okay with it – to be okay in the face of chaos – and you will fortify your mind and body.

RELATIONSHIP

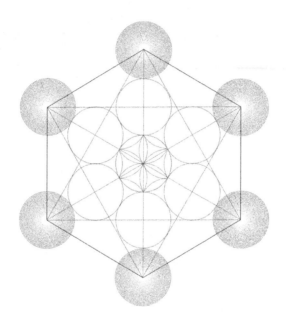

CHAPTER SEVEN

"To master a relationship is all about you... If you are aware that no one else can make you happy and that happiness is the result of love coming out of you, this becomes the greatest mastery of love."

Don Miguel Ruiz, The Mastery of Love

IN BUILDING RELATIONSHIPS, I think it is invaluable to recognize and understand the journeys of those who left lasting impressions, particularly the kinds of impressions that I have spent my life trying to overcome.

When my brothers and I were kids, my stepdad shared many stories about his own childhood. My mother told us stories too. Jack's childhood reflected in the relationships he built with me and my brothers.

In 2003 I visited the orphanages in Edinburgh with Jack and his younger brother, Terry. All of them. Many of the stories I heard as a child were fleshed out during that visit.

This was the stage when I forgave Jack for any residual resentment. I had worked on forgiveness over the years but this sealed the deal.

1951

It was Christmas Eve, and Jack was six years old. But he wasn't drifting off to sleep with visions of sugarplums in his head. He was staring up at the drab grey building in horror. This orphanage had a bad reputation. He wasn't sure exactly what happened here, but whatever it was, he wanted no part of it. It seemed he didn't have a choice.

His mom was a whore. If he didn't understand exactly at his young age exactly what that meant, he got the broad stroke of it. Strange men came in and out of the flat and disappeared into the bedroom with his mother. After they left, sometimes they would get food. But not always.

Things were getting worse and worse. The Scots always had a

reputation as being tough as nails, but the Depression and then the war had made Edinburgh gray and broken.

Times were hard and life was cheap. Jack's mother was pushing 30 and losing the luster of youth, and she could no longer feed the three mouths she had brought into the world. And so, instead of carols and presents, Jack and his brothers got the orphanage for Christmas that year. Tens of millions of people had gone to their deaths in bullets and gas and flames during the war, and the hardships of a few young boys in a cold, drab corner of Scotland were of little concern to anyone. The priests who ran the place operated with impunity.

Beatings were just a natural part of life. Psychological and emotional torture was to be expected. Without the church, these boys would have nothing. They would starve and die. They should praise Christ for their blessings. They could never pay back what had been given to them, but their labor, their love, their obedience, and their blood would be small offerings of thanks.

It was forbidden to own anything. All material things were given over to the church willingly with an open heart. But even before he was old enough to read, Jack knew he had to squirrel something away for himself and his brothers if they were going to survive. Every orphanage or jail or commune or other social institution creates an economy of its own. Services rendered. Items traded. Currency created.

Jack was bright and tough and thrifty. Despite warnings from the priests not to, he had stashed farthings and halfpennies away when he could come by them. The priests had surprise inspections from time to time and could easily find contraband stashed in mattresses and stuffed into shoes, but Jack was not so careless. He also knew there were spies in their midst – boys who would report back to the priests in exchange for certain privileges – so he never shared his hiding spot with anyone, not even his brothers.

But when he was 12, he was somehow found out. He came in from an afternoon of yard work, fingers tingling from the cold. He was tired and hungry, looking forward to a plate of beans and a good night's sleep. When he came into the room, he knew immediately neither of those things was in store for him on this night.

Four priests stood by his bed. The cloth bag he had stuffed his money into was on the pillow, the coins scattered on the sheet. He stopped dead in his tracks, but it was too late. Two of the older boys stepped up behind him. They were both 16 and he was only 12. He didn't stand a chance.

The whole dorm was assembled in the great hall. Usually, they'd be sitting on the long wooden benches eating bread and beans, but not tonight. They stood in straight rows, eyes front, arms at their sides. No fire burned in the fireplace. The room was cold and grey and somber.

"When a boy is baptized and receives the grace of Christ, he is saved," Father Seamus announced at last.

"He should give his life to Christ for the blessings he has received," he continued.

"Wouldn't you agree?" he asked, looking hard around the room. Every boy nodded his head and murmured his agreement.

"Aye, Father!" some of the more pious boys yelled out, to show their support. Father Seamus smiled.

"Some boys, however, forget their blessings. Like Judas, they betray their Lord," he said, lifting his arms to heaven.

"Judas stands before you tonight," he continued, pointing at Jack. All the boys stared at him, a mixture of pity and contempt on their faces.

"He has betrayed you. He has betrayed us all. But worst of all, he has betrayed Christ." Several of the boys hissed, right on cue.

"Strip him," Father Seamus said to the two younger priests who stood behind him at each elbow.

Roughly they seized him as two more priests came forward. They ripped his shirt away and cut the pants with scissors. In less than a minute, Jack stood naked at the front of the hall staring at a hundred sets of eyes that were filled with hate and horror.

"The Lord is not slack concerning his promise, as some men count slackness; but is long-suffering usward, not willing that any should perish, but that all should come to repentance," Father Seamus said, picking up a thick leather strap from the table beside him and holding it aloft for all to see.

"Be not deceived; God is not mocked: for whatsoever a man soweth, that shall he also reap."

And with that, the beating started. Father Seamus was meticulous, making sure to lash nearly every square inch of this pre-pubescent boy; across his legs and back, down his torso. And when at last the boy collapsed on the hard stone floor and curled into a ball, he lashed the bottoms of his feet, reciting verse after verse from the bible to justify the righteousness of his actions.

The next day, Jack was sent to live at another orphanage. He would never see his younger brother alive again.

1980

One morning, my stepfather Jack kicked my bed and said, "Get up and pack your things." Shawn, Jesse, and I sat up in our beds, wiping the sleep out of our eyes.

"What time is it?" I asked.

Jesse started to cry. He was only 10 years old, but somehow, he knew our lives were about to change – and not for the better.

Jack banged on the wall outside our door. "Shut up and start packing," he yelled, "or I'll come in there and give you something to cry about."

Shawn, who was 16, knew that wasn't an idle threat. Shawn was the toughest kid at school, and even the older kids wouldn't mess with him, but Jack could reduce him to tears with a combination of emotional humiliation and leather. Once the beatings started, Jack wouldn't give up until Shawn bawled. It might take two hours, but eventually even my older brother would crack.

"Shut the fuck up," Shawn hissed at Jesse. Nobody wanted to start this day with a beating. Jesse grew quiet, but the tears still streamed down his face.

Two hours later, we were all stuffed into the station wagon. My real father lived on a commune in a remote corner of Connecticut. We hadn't seen him in three or four years, and he had never been anything but a stranger to us. My mother smoked cigarettes in the front seat and explained to us that we were going to live with him now.

The FBI had just nabbed Jack with 10 pounds of weed, and family life with them was now impossible. We didn't know it yet but Jack planned to skip the country rather than face the U.S. justice system. He was going back to Scotland, where he had immigrated from nearly 30 years earlier. As it turned out, my mother would follow close behind.

We arrived at the commune in the heat of the day. It was a ramshackle cluster of hastily built huts and makeshift tents that encircled a small house in a clearing.

Women planted flowers in the garden around the house while two men repaired a gutter that had collapsed at one corner.

Jack sat in the driver's seat and kept the engine running as my mother kissed Shawn and me goodbye. Jesse sobbed in the back seat. He was Jack's son and was going with them – like it or not. After a few minutes, my mom got back into the car, and the three of them disappeared down the dirt road through the trees.

People started to come out of their tents and shacks or through the woods. All eyes were on these two strange boys, clustered in the center of the commune with sacks and pillowcases full of their belongings.

A grizzled-looking man emerged from one of the larger shacks. He was barefoot and bare-chested and had a wild look in his eye. His skin was a deep amber color, as if he'd spent his whole life baking in the sun. He had a hatchet in his hand, and as he approached, Shawn clenched his fists, ready for an attack.

"Shawn," said the old man to my brother, then he looked at me. "Troy," he nodded. And then I realized this wild-looking man in front of us was my father, James.

"What the fuck are you doing here?" he asked. "Mom said we're living here now," Shawn said.

A group of about 20 people had appeared on all sides. Everyone stared at us.

"How's that supposed to happen?" I asked. "Where are we supposed to go to school?" "There ain't no school here," my father said, spitting tobacco on the grass at my feet. "No shit," I said.

A man came out of the house and stood silently on the porch. He wore a pressed, white shirt and crisp, black slacks. Unlike everyone else who was barefoot, he had polished black shoes on his feet. He had a stern look, and I couldn't help but notice every adult bowed his or her head in his direction.

What was this place?

"Jack got nabbed for selling weed," Shawn said, as if that would explain everything. "So," my father grunted.

"So they can't keep us anymore."

My father blinked but nothing else. Silence, except for the hum of birds and locusts.

I looked at Shawn. "We can't live here," I said. He rolled his eyes and said nothing, but he didn't have to. I knew what he was thinking. "No shit, Sherlock."

The man on the porch came down the steps and approached, limping as quickly as his stiff frame would allow. He didn't even look at us kids.

"Get your fucking kids out of here," he barked at my father. "Not in five minutes but right fucking now!"

"Yes sir," he said, bowing and backing away. He grabbed my arm hard in his left hand and took Shawn by the wrist with his right. His calloused skin felt like a steel vise.

"C'mon," he ordered and dragged us toward a '74 Ford Econoline parked under a tarp stretched between some trees not far away. Soon we were on the highway, barreling back to where we had come from, although there was no "home" for us to go to anymore.

Shawn had a girlfriend and wanted to be dropped off at her house, so that's where we went next. He grabbed his stuff out of the back and slammed the door extra hard for emphasis. He turned and walked away, not saying a word. I could understand how he could hate Jack for this, but he seemed to be just as mad at me. No tearful goodbye. No "good luck" or "I'll see you soon." Just the back of his denim jacket as he walked away from the wreckage of our family.

My buddy Tom lived in a big house with lots of extra room. His parents were pretty easy-going, and I'd stayed at his house for weeks at a time before.

"Take a left," I said as we sped down the street.

"Right here," I pointed. My father careened around the corner and stepped on the gas. "Slow down, you're going to miss it," I said, pointing to the street as we passed it by. "Turn around," I said, pointing back in the other direction.

Something in the old man snapped. He slammed on the brakes

and turned to me with murder in his eyes. My stepfather had looked at me countless times in the same way, and nine times out of ten it was followed by a smack across the face. I braced myself. But before I knew it, he was out of the van. He threw open the back door and hurled my stuff into the ditch.

"Get out," he said. I didn't dare disobey.

My Kiss albums littered the ditch, strewn from the pillowcase my father had thrown there. As I slid *Love Gun* back into its sleeve, he showered me with gravel as he peeled out and sped back to the commune. My arm veins were popping as I carried the two heavy pillowcases – one stuffed with all my clothes and the other with my record collection – and trudged toward Tom's house. I cried along the way but did my best to dry my eyes before I got there. I didn't want to let on to anyone that I wasn't tough. I could handle anything life threw my way.

This was a milestone in my upbringing. These events were instrumental in changing my life: one moment I was a kid, the next I was on my own, fending for myself.

In the end these were the low times, the negative experiences that shaped my limbic system, my reptilian brain, that helped me navigate life in terms of survival. It was that moment when I found myself alone on the side of the road that hardened me, and gave me the tools to survive on my own as a teenager. More importantly, however, is looking back at those low times, those formative moments, and recognizing that while those were the trades of survival in my youth, they were no longer effective in my 20s, 30s, 40s, etc.

2006

I was in the Peruvian forest, breathing the clean air and feeling invigorated. My experience with ayahuasca had been life changing. The medicine was working. But the previous night, I had awoken from a vivid dream with my heart pounding in my chest.

We were skating on the lake in Connecticut, Shawn, Jesse, and I. Jesse was showing off his new skates. He'd sprint across the ice, then do a hockey stop, spraying snow and slush up into Shawn's face. Normally, Shawn would pound him for this, but Jesse was a surprisingly fast skater, and Shawn – who was a natural at most sports – was slow and awkward on the ice.

"Hit him again," I yelled, egging Jesse on. Jesse must have been about eight – before the family split apart, and he was as happy as I can ever remember seeing him.

"Yes sir!" He saluted, then spun around and sprinted across the ice.

"Try it and you die!" warned Shawn. He packed a snowball and got ready for the assault. But suddenly Jesse disappeared. There was a muffled cry, then nothing.

Shawn and I looked at each other, and then took off across the ice. I could see the hole where Jesse had gone through, and slid up to it on my belly, Pete Rose style. Jesse was there, under the water, a look of panic on his face. He was reaching wildly for something to grab onto as he sunk into the cold black depths.

"Jesse!" I screamed, reaching for him.

The water was frigid, and my arm burned like it was on fire. Shawn finally skated up awkwardly.

"Grab my ankles," I told him, and started to slide the upper half of my body into the water.

Jesse reached for my arm, but he was already too far down. I lurched forward, thinking I might be able to snatch him but something was holding me back. Shawn had done what I told him to, and now I was stuck. Jesse kicked wildly, a look of sheer terror in his eyes as an air bubble escaped his throat. Our fingers touched, but before I could grab him he was gone. I was being pulled up out of the water, my face burning from the cold.

"Jesse!" I sat up in my cot, frantic. Jesse was in trouble. I knew it.

Jesse had been struggling with heroin for years. The last time I saw him, he was a shell of his former self. That cocky strut of his twenties was gone. The twinkle in his eye was no more. He was barely into his 30s, but he looked twice that old. His skin was pale. He stunk.

I was so afraid that my dream had been a premonition, that when I heard him croak, "hello," I almost cried.

"Jesse, is that you?" "Yeah. Who's this?"

"It's Troy." Silence. "Your brother." "Hey Troy, what's up?"

"I am in Peru," I said. Another long silence. "Perdue?"

"No...Peru. South America. The Amazon man!" "Seriously? What are you doing there?"

"It's a long story," I told him. "And these long-distance calls are expensive, so I can't talk for long. But it's amazing here, and I want you to come here with me."

"To the Amazon? What the fuck, Troy?"

"Trust me, little brother. You'll love it here. Knowing you, you'll never want to go back." Silence.

"I am going to bring you down here. My treat. It'll change your life, I swear." "They got methadone down there?" he asked.

"Even better! They got ayahuasca." "What's that?"

"You'll see. I think it can help you. And there's a medicine man here I want you to meet." "I don't know, Troy."

"Listen, we'll talk more when I get stateside. I am going to be down here a few more weeks. I am filming some amazing footage, bro. You're gonna love it here, I promise."

More silence.

"I gotta go. Take care of yourself, and I'll see you soon, okay?" Silence.

"Jesse?"

"Yeah Troy. See you soon."

I slept better after that. Some nights I would dream of Jesse and me exploring the Amazon jungle together. He was strong and healthy in my dreams. The ayahuasca had cured him, and the poison was out of his veins. He smiled again, and that twinkle was back in his eye. I felt a sense of pride that, for once, I was able to help him.

But not all dreams come true. By the time I arrived back in the U.S. I got word that Jesse had died of an overdose. I never saw my little brother again. One month later, Little Troy was born – the spitting image of his uncle.

2018

Resentment is toxic. It's like drinking poison and expecting the other person to get sick. Divorce put all my philosophies to the test.

I am a humble, kind, and gentle man.

Words are easy. Actions are hard. The divorce was final, but it didn't feel like the end of anything. Uri and I had brought two souls into this world and, like it or not, we were linked together forever.

And we still fought about how to raise the kids. I was a disciplinarian. She was permissive. Or nurturing. Pick your verb. When it was my time to have them, they'd come over to my house and we'd go camping, or hang out at the beach, or ride bikes, or swim in the ocean. Everybody had chores at dinnertime. Athena would chop the herbs and sweep the floor. Little Troy did the dishes and took out the trash.

One time, Uri came to pick them up and asked them to wait in the car while we had "an adult conversation."

"They're not your maids, Troy," she said. "Why are you always making them do chores? They're too young."

"First of all...bullshit. And secondly BULLSHIT! Who are you to tell me they're too young to help with dinner?"

The only thing "adult" about our conversations was the language. It was unproductive and escalating. We could have waged World War III on each other, but to what end? Total annihilation?

No. I wanted peace. True peace and forgiveness. But the strategies that worked for me in my 20s, 30s, and 40s weren't working in my 50s.

I had to somehow get past all the emotional baggage I had carried for so many years. I needed to learn to forgive. To view my relationships in a positive light. To come to understand that all of my experiences were done *for* me, not *to* me.

So once again I turned to the gratitude journal. I wanted to focus on my relationships, to learn to be grateful even for those things that were painful. My single prayer was peace and harmony.

I am grateful for the mistakes my family made that resulted in us breaking up as they taught me the value of family.

When Athena and Troy stay over, I sometimes watch them sleep for hours. These two amazing souls came into my life and blessed me more than I could ever hope for. Little Troy not only looks like his uncle, but also has so many of the same mannerisms. I think he must be the reincarnated soul of my brother.

I am grateful for the emotional abuse I endured as it helped me focus on being a better father.

I used to hate my stepfather. I'd lay awake after a beating and dream of all the horrible ways I'd make him suffer if I had the power to. After visiting him in 2003 and touring the orphanages with him; after he told me all the terrible things that had happened there, I actually felt sorry for him. He had suffered so much physical and psychological abuse as a child, it was a wonder he could even function. He showed me a dimension of a father I never wanted to be. I am not a perfect father – far from it. But my children are interested, and interesting. They aren't allowed to be rude or vain or selfish, but they aren't allowed to take shit from anyone either. I could not be the father I am without living the life I've lived.

I am grateful for growing up on the street as it made me strong.

Each time life knocked me down, I got back up. Depression, disease, death, and sorrow had come into my life, but providence had prepared me at an early age to take care of myself.

I am grateful for my father dropping me off on the side of the street as it taught me how to be resilient.

When it was time to sink or swim, I swam. Years later, I asked my father what he was feeling when he left me there on the side of the road. He couldn't look me in the eye or articulate any meaningful answer. I hated him for what he had done, and I hated him even more for his lack of remorse. Even as my spiritual journey led me away from darkness and into the light, I held the resentment in the pit of my stomach. But now I began to see how even the lowest moments had shaped me. Who would I be without them? And who among us gets to choose where the shadow falls across their lives?

I am grateful for my upbringing as it helped me understand that everyone has a shadow, including me.

Perfection doesn't exist. We are all perfectly imperfect, just the way

God intended us to be. My mother and father are flawed, as am I. My children aren't perfect, but I love them with all my heart, even as I sometimes fail them.

I am grateful I could witness my stepfather's anger so I can understand myself better and heal myself.

My stepfather used to beat the shit out of me. He was angry all the time. Angry at his boss. Angry at his wife. Angry at life. And who can blame him, having the shitty childhood he had? I would be angry too. But I saw what anger did to him. How it ate him up inside. He tried to wear his anger like armor, but it crushed him under its weight and poisoned everyone closest to him.

I am grateful for my grandmother not approving of my choice to move to Los Angeles and become an actor. The negativity provided an atmosphere for me to prove her wrong with a stronger resolve to be successful.

My grandmother and I have always engaged in emotional Aikido. Maybe she knew the only sure way to get me to do something was to tell me not to do it. Or maybe she just thought I'd fail. I have to admit, it was a solid bet. But her disapproval was a driving force without which I may not have succeeded.

I am grateful for being locked up in juvenile hall as it taught me the importance of freedom.

My spiritual journey is a journey of liberation, yet the paradox eluded me until my 50th year. Nothing we do is by ourselves. We are in a symbiotic relationship with everything, and everyone. And when you understand that you are never really free of anything, you'll be free from everything.

I am grateful for my troubles with drugs and alcohol, as they led me to meditation.

Meditation first showed me the veils over my eyes, and then taught me how to pull them back. Meditation has brought peace into my mind, which has brought peace into my body. Healthy mind, healthy body. Strong mind, strong body.

I am grateful for all my trials and tribulations, as they provided the opportunity for me to always go deeper!

I am the captain of my life and will sail my soul to the ports of my choice. And, when gale-force winds try to blow me back from my destination and my skill to drive ahead is at its limit, I've been shown new ways. Ayahuasca, 5-MEO-DMT, and other plant medicines are tools in the toolkit to open the mind, to see new possibilities. And once the possibilities are conceived, they can be achieved.

I am grateful for the emotional abuse I endured, as it created stagnation and indigestion in my gut, which led me on an endless search to optimize my body and mind, giving me the knowledge and wisdom to help others.

With me, it's always about the gut. I was constipated my entire adult life. Life literally was not flowing through me. But step by step, year by year, I was taught how to heal myself. I had come so far. So many veils had been lifted from my eyes. What was once an impressionistic blur of shapes and colors had come into focus, but a thin layer of mist remained. And now I had the key to peel it away and see with truly clear eyes. And the answer was so simple.

Forgiveness.

I forgave my father for leaving me by the side of the road. I forgave my mother for leaving me with my father. I forgave Jack for the beatings. I forgave Jesse for dying and Shawn for not loving me the way I wanted an older brother to love me. I forgave Uri for making me second-guess myself as a father, for trying to emasculate me as a husband.

I forgave myself for all my failings. For the drugs and the alcohol. For the DUI. For not saving Jesse. For holding onto the darkness for so long.

I let all the anger and resentment drain out of me, and the last wisp of fog blew away with the breeze. And now everything was in perfect balance.

And yet...there on the horizon, I can see something new. Something big and important. And I know now that the last veil will never be lifted. There will always be more to see, and learn, and know. It is a trap to think you've ever arrived, because that will stop you from moving forward. And that leads to stagnation.

But where I go from here will not be on a ship by myself. My family will be with me, and my friends too. And more than that, everyone on this planet is on my ship. I am in a relationship with the All, and the All with me.

As above, so below. Our relationships are part of our DNA, woven into the very fabric of our beings. When our relationships are troubled, our bodies become inflamed. But when our relationships are healthy, so can we be.

Building Your Relationship Pillar

You are not alone. You are connected to everyone, and everyone is connected to you. The relationships you form with friends and family help guide your path in life. They help you build bridges to overcome obstacles. And they can also be the source of your biggest roadblocks.

Here are some tips for building your Relationship Pillar:

Food, Friends, and Family

Some of my fondest memories of life are sitting around the table with friends and family. Sharing a good meal with the people I love is one of my greatest joys. Food nourishes us when we're hungry, comforts us when we're feeling low, and heals us when we are sick. Sharing a meal is one of the great ways to say "I love you." Make time in your life to share a meal with those you love.

Grace

Even though I'm not a religious person in the traditional sense, saying grace before a meal is a great way to build relationships. This variation on the gratitude journal lets me share my gratitude with those I have a meal with. Take a minute or two before the meal to tell those you love how thankful you are for them, then give them the opportunity to do the same. It's a beautiful way to begin a meal.

Travel

Whether taking a walk in the park or traveling to some distant location, getting into nature with my friends and family is one of my favorite things to do. Riding bikes to the farmer's market, paddle-boarding in the bay, camping under the redwoods, summiting a peak... these are great ways to build relationships and connect with nature.

Forgiveness

Relationships that exist over a long period of time will experience darkness. Words may be spoken that should not have been. Some words that should be spoken are left unsaid. Fights may happen. Disappointments or even trauma may occur. Don't let your issues freeze in your tissues. Resentment is toxic. If you can find forgiveness in your heart, you can release old traumas. Relationships can be beautiful, messy things. They can be a source of comfort and grace if you let them. Learn to forgive past grievances. If you can do this, your relationships will grow stronger.

WATER

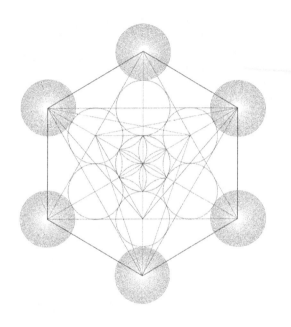

CHAPTER EIGHT

"The cell is immortal. It is merely the fluid in which it floats that degenerates. Renew this fluid at regular intervals, give the cells what they require for nutrition, and as far as we know, the pulsation of life can go on forever."

Dr. Alexis Carrell, Nobel Prize winner

Standing Rock

IN DECEMBER 2016, I found myself protesting the North Dakota pipeline at Standing Rock. I went there to show my support for the protection of all water globally and the solutions I propose for our sustainable future: free energy, self-care education, the gift economy, contributionism, and permaculture. I did not go there as a victim. I am not interested in ascribing blame to "they" or "others" as the cause of problems in the world. We are collectively responsible for the world we have created, and therefore we must collectively come up with the solutions to these problems.

I fly on a planes and drive in cars, and I am grateful that I can do these things. I am a citizen of the modern world and I enjoy the conveniences and luxuries this world provides me. I love to travel and see the world, and I hope for a future in which we can travel with zero pollution, but I understand that is not our reality today.

I went with love and reverence for the earth in my heart. I believe clean air, water, and soil should be the common human heritage. They are what make life here on earth hospitable and possible for us. I want to leave this world better than I found it, and I want my children, and their children, to grow up in a world where clean air, water, and soil is a reality.

I listened to the local Lakota people tell their stories. I wanted to learn more about their connection to the earth and to water. One evening, I sat around a campfire with about 20 other protesters as an elder told the Lakota creation story. I didn't record this on camera, so I will do my best to retell it as accurately as I can.

Lakota Creation Story

This is not the first world. Long ago, there was another world. In the beginning, that world was beautiful and the people were good. Everyone lived in peace. But it didn't last. The people became wicked and made the world ugly. The Creating Power grew angry. He began to sing and rain fell from the sky. His second song brought storms that ripped up trees and swelled the rivers. His third song brought floods and destruction, and his fourth song split the earth. The whole world was engulfed by the flood. All the people drowned. Only Kangi the crow survived.

Kangi flew and flew for days but could find no place to land. He cried out to the Creating Power, pleading for a place to rest. The Creating Power took pity on Kangi and decided to make a new world.

The Creating Power had a pipe bag filled with all of the animals in the world. He picked four animals that could stay underwater for a long time and sent them each to retrieve a lump of soil from beneath the floodwaters.

The loon was first to dive into the dark waters but was unable to reach the bottom. The otter tried next, but her strong webbed feet could not propel her deep enough. After her went the beaver, but he also failed. Finally, the turtle took a deep breath and disappeared into the dark waters. Turtle was gone so long that Kangi thought he had drowned. Just as Kangi was about to give up and fall into the water himself, Turtle appeared with a splash. Mud filled his claws and the cracks in his shell.

The Creating Power took the mud in his hands and began to sing. Then he spread the mud on the water and made a place just big enough for himself and Kangi. Next, he took two eagle feathers and shook them over the mud until the earth spread out in every direction. Filled with sadness for the dry land, he wept, and his tears became the streams, lakes, and oceans of the world. He named the new land Turtle Continent to honor the turtle that provided the mud from which it is formed.

The Creating Power took animals of all kinds from his pipe bag and populated the earth, then formed men and women from the red, white, yellow, and black soil. He gave the new people his sacred pipe and told them to live by it. He gave them the whole, beautiful world and promised that all would be well if they lived in harmony. Then he told them of the fate of the people of the old world and told them this new world could be destroyed again if they made it ugly.

Water

Water is the source of all life on earth. Life on this planet originated in water billions of years ago and without water every living thing on this planet would die. Water is the most common substance on earth. It is the only element that can exist in three forms (solid, liquid, and gas), and it is the only element that expands when frozen, and contracts when heated. Every other element known to man does the exact opposite.

Why?

The truth is, no one knows. The mystery of life on this planet is – in part – the mystery of water. And while immortality is probably not a viable option for our bodies, longevity certainly is. I want to live a long and healthy life, and I'd be willing to guess you do too. So let's talk about water and hydration.

The Solution to Pollution Is Dilution

In simplest terms, your body converts food into energy and filters contaminants out. Water is an essential ingredient in this process.

These contaminants can come from the water we drink, the air we breathe, and the food we eat. The purer the water, air, and food you take in, the better your body will be at creating energy and filtering waste.

Unfortunately, in the world we live in, your body is being besieged by contaminants and is forced to work harder and harder to keep up. Municipal water systems that contain chlorine, fluoride, and maybe even lead can make it a challenge to drink clean, pure water. Highly processed foods that are full of glyphosate, GMOs, and chemical additives compromise our natural digestive and immune systems.

Polluted air coats our skin, infects our respiratory system, and wreaks havoc on our health.

Water can be our biggest ally in getting rid of the many contaminants that assail us every day. I like to say, "The solution to pollution is dilution!"

By 2016, I was putting the 9 Pillars into balance. My legacy was crystal clear. I had cut gluten out of my diet. I removed inflammatory agents like soy, corn, and wheat. I cleaned phytic acid out of my system, removing the nuts, grains, and seeds that carry it. My nutrition was right on point.

I was sleeping well and moving as well as I ever had in my lifetime. Breath work was keeping my head clear and emotions in check. My thinking was positive and strong. My relationships were deep and loving, and I was truly connecting with nature in meaningful ways.

But, as I have mentioned a number of times, with me, all things go back to my gut. I have struggled with constipation my whole adult life, and I knew I had to conquer this demon once and for all. I was still using herbs to maintain my regularity, and I decided I needed to finally do away with that crutch.

At that time, Dr. Pee Pee Shivambu was coming over to my house and teaching me breath work. We also talked about his urine therapy. I had been doing urine therapy myself for the last 15 years. It's biofeedback. Real hair of the dog. Our bodies are self-healing miracles. I drank my middle stream every morning. When I got up, I'd pee a little out, put some in a cup, then pee out the rest. I was also using aged urine topically, to restore and rejuvenate my skin.

But Dr. Pee Pee Shivambu taught me lots of other ways to use it. He taught me to age and ferment it. And he taught me how to use the aged urine for enemas.

I was amazed at the parasites that came out of me. Once, I turned around to see little square jellyfish-looking creature in the toilet. It had a soft little hook coming out of it, and it was the weirdest thing I've ever seen.

Metaphysically, constipation is a sign that I wasn't letting life flow through me. I'd battled it my entire adult life. It was my curse. But it was also my gift. It drove me to go deeper and deeper into my spiritual journal to find an answer. And then finally, I had a breakthrough.

The aged urine enemas finally healed my gut. I felt life begin to flow through me.

My gut brain had been infected by strange parasites for as long as I can remember. Maybe it was the antibiotics I took as a kid. They were harsh, wiping out all bacteria, good and bad, indiscriminately. They dropped an atomic bomb on my gut, unleashing monsters from the deep.

They say traumatic childhood experiences can freeze into your flesh. A rape. A beating. A humiliation. They can leave traces of themselves in your cells for years.

I don't know where my gut demons came from, but when I finally was rid of them, everything changed. For the first time in my life, I felt like everything was in balance. I was authentically living my philosophy. I was *RippedAt50*.

But I get it. Gut issues may not haunt you like they did me. And urine therapy isn't for everyone. But there are lots of other ways you can dilute the pollution from your body through good hydration.

Quality

The fact is that your body is about 70% water. The better the quality of the water you put into your body, the better your body will operate. Natural water is the best, but since we've contaminated most of the water on earth, that may not be a realistic option for you. Most likely, you will need to drink purified water.

Structuring and re-mineralizing purified water with a pinch of sea salt or ionic elements will help the water's mineral balance.

Water is the most powerful solvent on earth. In other words, more chemical compounds dissolve in water than any other element we know of. This is what makes water essential for life. It also means you need to pay attention to the delivery system between the source of the water and your body.

As the people of Flint, Michigan know, lead in pipes can dissolve and contaminate a water supply. Water can also leach toxins out of other materials Water that sits in plastic for a long time, especially when sunlight is present, can dissolve the chemical elements that make up plastic and introduce toxins and xenoestrogens into your system.

Xenoestrogens are similar enough to estrogen to confuse your body. They have been the source of numerous scientific studies over the past 10 years, with many studies finding hard evidence of adverse health effects on humans. Xenoestrogens can bind themselves to receptor sites and act as "false messengers" that can disrupt reproduction and other natural processes. And as much as I like to get in touch with my feminine side, ingesting unwanted xenoestrogens is not my preferred method.

Personally, I like to drink water out of glass. I get natural spring water delivered to my home in glass bottles. It is expensive, but hey, I am worth it!

Artesian spring water is filtered through the earth slowly for thousands of years and becomes naturally mineralized in the process. I sometimes add additional minerals to make sure my body has what it needs, including:

- Redmond clay
- Pure camu camu powder
- Celtic sea salt
- Herbs and superfoods grown in mineral-rich soil

I've also installed a quadruple filtration system in my home. This reverse-osmosis system filters out many of the contaminants in my municipal water supply, because who wants a tall glass of pharmaceutical drugs, feces, urine, and toilet paper? Not me!

Filtering your shower is also a good idea. If you've followed the work of Erin Brockovich (or seen the movie starring Julia Roberts), you have seen how toxic industrial waste can seep into community water supplies and cause serious disease. And, if you've followed what is going on in Flint, you know that many of our cities have decaying infrastructures that could put your health at risk. Protect yourself and your family by being more conscious about the water put onto and into your body.

Quantity

It is also important to think about how much water you drink. I drink half my body weight (lbs.) in ounces of water daily. I weigh about 170 lbs., so I divide that in half (85) and drink that many ounces of water every day. This is a general guideline and may go up if I am exercising more, or if it's really hot and I am sweating a lot.

Water is a great detoxifier as well as a daily necessity. When you're looking at balancing nutrition, your body must be able to metabolize materials and make them available in your blood. Water and minerals are key.

Water is the source of all life on earth. Giving your body the right amount of the highest-quality water you can is essential for health. Here are a few tips to build your Water Pillar.

Delivery System

In a perfect world, you could drink fresh, clean water directly in nature. Unfortunately, we've contaminated most of the water on earth, so you're not likely to have that reality. You will probably get your water through other delivery systems. For most, that means a municipal water supply. Even in good systems, the potential for trace amounts of pharmaceutical drugs, feces, urine, and toilet paper are there. And in worst-case scenarios (like Flint, MI) much more dangerous poisons can be introduced. I have two systems I use: one for the water I drink, and another for household use.

Drinking Water

Drinking the purest water possible is just as important as eating the highest-quality natural or organic foods. It is essential! For my drinking water, I have artesian spring water delivered in glass containers. Artesian spring water is filtered through the earth for thousands of years and becomes naturally mineralized in the process. When considering the extra cost of glass containers over plastic, remember that water is the most powerful solvent on earth. Water that sits in plastic, especially where light is present, can introduce xenoestrogens. As the name implies, xenoestrogens come from external sources, but are similar enough to estrogen to confuse your body. Xenoestrogens can disrupt reproduction and other natural processes.

- **How much to drink** – On average, drink half your body weight (lbs.) in ounces of water daily.

  o Example: If you weigh 100 pounds, drink 50 ounces of water daily.

- **Supplements** – I sometimes add the following to make sure my body gets the minerals it needs:

    o   Redmond clay

    o   Pure camu camu powder

    o   Celtic sea salt

    o   Herbs and superfoods grown in mineral-rich soil

Household Water

The quality of the water that you put on your body (in baths and showers) is also important. Our skin has a higher absorption rate than the linings of our stomach, and we need to be mindful of what we allow ourselves to come into contact with. I've installed a quadruple filtration system in my home. This reverse-osmosis system filters out many of the contaminants in my municipal water supply to help keep my family safe.

The Solution to Pollution is Dilution

In simplest terms, your body converts food into energy and filters contaminants out. Water is an essential ingredient. Water can be one of the most effective tools you can use to keep your body as clean and healthy as possible. Start with the highest-quality water you can get.

NATURE

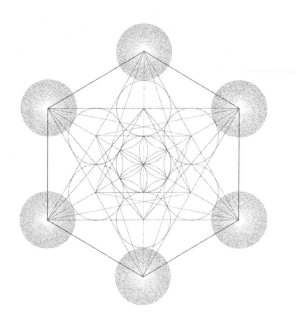

CHAPTER NINE

*"Natural forces within us
are the true healers of disease."*

Hippocrates

WHEN I WAS 13, we lived on a lake in Connecticut. I spent the summers swimming with my brothers, and in the winter, we'd skate on the ice. The back of the property opened onto a forest that stretched for miles and miles in all directions. The power company cut a path through that forest for the high-voltage lines, and my brothers and I would hike along those lines for hours, rarely seeing another human being.

Krissy L. lived on her family's farm along those lines, and I'd sneak out at night to see her. Finding my way by moonlight, or even with the help of fireflies, we'd rendezvous in the horse barn, climb up into the loft, and make out.

The following summer, things started to get more serious. I was 14, and my hormones were raging. Krissy's parents had gone out of town, and we had planned to get together for a big night. I'd even bragged to my little brother Jesse how wet I was going to make Krissy. He didn't know what that meant, but it sounded pretty good to him!

Unfortunately, I got in trouble and I was grounded.

I lay there sweating on my sheets, listening to the thrum of cicadas outside my window, feeling my heartbeat heavy in my chest. I was desperate to see her, as only a horny 14-year-old boy could be. I knew that if I got caught, my stepdad would beat the living shit out of me, but after three hours I couldn't take it anymore.

I crept across the floor as quietly as I could, avoiding the loose floorboard that I knew would creak if I stepped on it. I took the screen out of my window and put it in my closet, then slowly – achingly slowly – I crept down the trellis. I could hear the ballgame on the TV in the living room and hear my stepdad curse the lousy pitching, so I knew he was still awake. If I got caught, I'd be dead.

I clung to the side of the house, waiting for the right moment.

Finally, the pitcher retired the side and the old man clapped his hands and let out, "It's about time!" Just then I leaped to the ground and rolled across the grass just like I'd seen Bruce Lee do.

I made my way out through the back of our property, but the night was so pitch black I couldn't see anything. I had neglected to bring a flashlight with me, but luckily I had a pack of matches in my pocket that helped me find my way.

When I finally made it to Krissy's house, my hormones were in overdrive. I was about to pop. Unfortunately, Krissy wasn't there. Instead, I found Krissy's little sister Kathy sitting on the front porch. Kathy told me some of the kids had taken their parents' car out for a joyride and crashed it in a ditch. No one was hurt, but the fender had fallen off and they were in deep trouble.

Obviously, this was not going to be my night. The evening just took a huge nosedive. Getting my ass kicked after sleeping with Krissy would've been worth it. Taking a beating with blue balls? Not so much. I sighed deeply, turned, and made my way toward home.

Hopefully, I could sneak back in without getting caught.

Back on the highway, the cops had arrived to investigate the crash, and it was just my luck to run smack into one at the end of Krissy's driveway.

"Who the hell are you?" the cop asked, shining his flashlight in my eyes. "Um..." I stalled.

Luckily just then a call came in on his radio, and when he turned to grab it, I ran. "Hey!" he called after me, but I was gone.

I was running wild through the woods, under the power lines. I couldn't see a thing, but I was too amped up to care about little details like that. I ran and ran until I thought my lungs would explode. My legs were on fire and felt as heavy as lead.

At one point, the power lines turned to the right, but it was so dark I didn't even notice. A few feet past the turn there was a steep ledge that dropped sharply down to a dirty little cattle pond. By the time I was on the slope, I knew it was too late, and I splashed face-first into the muck. I came up spluttering, peeling a slimy lily pad from my face.

Suddenly a flashlight hit me in the eyes. Dammit! How did that fat cop keep up with me for so long?

Then I heard the laughing and let out a sigh of relief. It was my brother Jesse and his friend Dale.

"Oh man," Jesse laughed. "That was classic! What the fuck are you doing, Troy?" "Some cop stopped me up on Route 6, so I just ran."

Dale and Jesse fell over laughing.

"I thought you said you were gonna make Krissy wet. Look who's wet now, dumbass!" Jesse roared.

Jesse, it seems, also snuck out of the house that night. He and Dale had gotten the story from Kathy before I had and were heading home when I went running past them in the dark.

"I hope dad didn't check our rooms," I said.

The smile faded from Jesse's face. "Let's get home before he does." We made it home at about 1:30 am and snuck back into the house without getting caught.

Later that summer, I lost my virginity to Krissy L. up in the loft of the horse barn. I guess you could say it was my first official "roll in the hay." I'll always remember my sexual awakening and running around in those woods that summer.

Whenever I close my eyes and think about my connection to nature, my mind inevitably wanders back to my youth in those innocent days before my family fell apart. Breathing the fresh air, walking for miles along the forest floor, smelling the fresh pine, and listening to the hum of insects and the whisper of wind in the trees. My connection with nature was innocent and joyous. I felt truly at peace in that forest.

Time and again throughout my life, in good times and in bad, my connection with nature has been crucial. At age 13, I took this connection for granted. At 54, my love for nature has grown infinitely more complex. And once in a while, just like my grandma, Mother Nature gives me a smack on the head when I get out of line.

One time a few years ago, I was camping in Yosemite. It was a Sunday afternoon, and the crowds were heading home. We had done a major hike the day before and had gotten up early to see the sunrise, so I wanted to catch a little power nap before dinner.

But Mother Nature had other plans for me that day. Now that all the people had cleared out, chipmunks took their opportunity to raid the trashcans for an afternoon snack.

A hawk circled overhead, so the chipmunks chattered and

chattered, alerting everyone in the clan as to the whereabouts of the predator in the sky. They would much rather eat lunch than be lunch.

As tired as I was, I just couldn't drown out the incessant chattering, and soon I found myself in the middle of the campsite yelling at those chipmunks.

"Why don't you just shut the fuck up?"

There was a fat chipmunk standing on a rock nearby, and he didn't much care for the tone of my voice.

Chatter chatter chatter. "What did you call me?"

CHATTER CHATTER CHATTER!

That's it! I am not going to take that from a rodent. I picked up a pinecone and threw it at him.

CHATTER CHATTER CHATTER CHATTER CHATTER CHATTER CHATTER

"Ah!!!! Beat it!" I threw another pinecone.

Now they were just laughing at me. How humiliating. I was so tired that I was yelling at chipmunks. The audacity of my ego!

I sat down under a giant redwood and leaned back against the rough bark. I needed to calm myself.

But the fat chipmunk was not done with me yet. He snuck around the other side of the tree and climbed up to some high branches hundreds of feet above me. He found the hardest pinecone he could find, plucked it from the tree, and aimed carefully.

Down, down, down the pinecone fell, picking up speed as it went until – BONK – it landed right on top of my head. If you've never had a pinecone dropped on your head from such a height, let me tell you, it hurts. A lot.

But I couldn't help but laugh as I rubbed the knot growing on the top of my skull. You have to respect even Mother Nature's smallest creatures.

As above, so below. This is the natural law of correspondence, and it applies to every pillar of my philosophy, perhaps most of all to nature. It is no coincidence that throughout the ages, writers and philosophers, poets and saints have all personified nature as our mother. Giver of life. Nurturer. Comforter. Protector.

Everything vital for life is provided by nature. Oxygen, water, and nutrition all flow from the grace of nature. And the health of our bodies and our minds cannot be separated from the health of our planet. My spiritual journey has brought me into closer and closer communion with our common mother. It has taught me a reverence and awe for the incredible gifts we are given so freely. It has taught me to use the tools that nature gives us to heal myself and to live in peace and harmony.

Nature is the first pillar and the last pillar. It is so fundamental to our wellbeing that discussing it should be totally unnecessary. But human beings are a curious lot. We can convince ourselves of almost anything, and in my lifetime, I've seen our species lose a lot of ground on this important subject.

Sadly, as our health and nutrition become more of a commodity, huge multinational conglomerates develop vested financial interest in selling us food products, misinformation, and half-truths. Even outright lies have become mainstream. Our nutritional choices are now determined by the advertising executives of massive corporations.

In some ways, we've made tremendous progress in science and medicine, fitness and nutrition. But, in other ways, we've gone backward. Sometimes we're told that we can "improve" on Mother Nature. As I apply the scientific method to my life, I approach "breakthrough" claims with the skepticism they deserve. In the chapter on nutrition, I wrote at length about glyphosate – the so-called "miracle" herbicide that was supposed to kill weeds while leaving our crops untouched. If you believe the marketing materials of the chemical company behind these products, crop yields improve and the food is perfectly safe for humans. But dig deeper, and the story is much more complicated. I believe these chemicals have infected our food system. I believe the food we put into our bodies has fundamentally changed, and it is having a catastrophic effect on our health.

There are other important ways that mass media and the corporatization of health is negatively influencing our relationship with nature.

Bacteria

Over the past 20 years, there has been a concerted effort to convince us that all bacteria are bad. Antibacterial sprays and soaps have been marketed as a way to keep us safe. The claim is that if you love your family and you want to protect them from harm, you need to kill all of the bacteria in your house and live in a sterile environment.

But this is a dangerous fallacy. It's an interesting paradox that humans are made up of about 10% human cells and 90% bacterial cells. And while there are some "bad" bacteria that can cause sickness and disease if given an opportunity to thrive, much of the bacteria that live inside us and on us are beneficial, even *essential* for good health. We have lived in a symbiotic relationship with these microbes since the dawn of humanity. They help us digest our food, clean our bodies of toxins, and kill dangerous invaders.

Antibiotics are another example of how our war against bacteria has become self-defeating. We are all-knowing, self-healing creatures of God. When our minds and bodies are healthy, Mother Nature provides us with all the tools we need to rid our systems of dangerous invaders. But sometimes, when our immune systems are compromised, bad bacteria can get the upper hand and lead to problems.

The term "antibiotic" in and of itself should make you stop and think. Translated from the Greek "anti" meaning against and "biotic" meaning life, antibiotics literally mean "against life." While I understand there are some legitimate uses for this tool, I also believe it is a blunt instrument that should be used rarely and with caution. Antibiotics can be like an atomic bomb. True, they can wipe out the enemy, but they can also reduce the "civilian" population to ashes at the same time.

How many people do you know who go running for antibiotics at the first sign of infection, as if it were a miracle cure? Beware! Many times, you're better off letting your immune system take care of the bad bacteria rather than carpet-bombing your entire system.

The Sun

Another of nature's miracles that has come under attack is the sun. We're told that radiation from the sun is harmful to our health and that science has the answer (in the form of sunscreen and UV-protection glasses). This, to me, is a dangerous narrative.

The fact is, life on earth is reliant on the sun. And while it is true that the incidence of skin cancer has skyrocketed, I believe this is mostly due to our changing relationship with nature rather than any inherent danger posed by the sun's rays.

We have been engineered over millennia to survive and thrive in our natural environment, and the sun is the cornerstone of that relationship. We know that certain plants thrive in harsh equatorial sunlight. Seaweed and some tropical plants, herbs, seeds, and berries produce incredible photochemistry out of this radiation. The more you flood your body with these types of nutrients, the more your skin responds.

Studies have also shown that indigenous people with massive exposure to sunlight have a low incidence of skin cancer. Dr. James Duke, a leading ethnobotanist who spent his life studying natural medicine and healing herbs, found that one plant, in particular, had a powerful protective quality against the radiation of the sun. He found that indigenous people living in the Amazon River basin who drank a tea made with local plants did not seem to get sunburned. Again, while science scrambles to explain why, I believe their diets and their natural relationship with the sun protects them from the harmful rays that might otherwise cause skin cancer.

I also believe that, like glyphosate in our food, chemicals that we slather on our skin to protect us from the sun may be doing more harm than good. Our skin has a higher absorption rate than the linings of our stomach, and we need to be mindful of what we allow ourselves to come into contact with.

No one wants to damage his or her skin, but the sun provides so many positive benefits for our health it seems ridiculous to focus on the potential negative aspects. The question becomes how do you get sun exposure without damaging your skin? If you practice internal purification and clean eating and flood your body with micro-nutrition with fresh-squeezed juice and herbs, as well as making sure you have low stress levels, then some sunlight can be beneficial. It is about using cognition, intelligence, and intuition as a guide to how much sunlight is the best for your body.

Yes, the sun can damage you. But before you slather toxic chemicals all over your body, read the ingredients. Those ingredients may clog your pores. The skin is the largest organ in the body; and clogging it up with toxic compounds is not the answer. Eating a diet rich in fat-soluble chemicals may be a recipe for skin cancer. I personally don't use sunscreen, but if you feel sunscreen is right for you, take a close look at the ingredients to avoid ingesting potentially toxic elements into your system—it is safe to avoid any ingredient you cannot pronounce. There are many nontoxic sunscreen options available.

Sunglasses may also be counterproductive. By blocking the part of the light spectrum that drives your endocrine system, you may be robbing yourself of essential chemicals your body needs to protect you against radiation. That is the reason I rarely, if ever, wear sunglasses. In fact, I believe that light is a form of nutrition. Light is biophotonic energy, and we are energy beings. The way we get our biophotonic energy is through the closed organic cycle. The closed organic cycle works like this: Plants convert energy from the sun into energy through photosynthesis. This process uses chlorophyll, which is known as plant blood. Chlorophyll has the exact molecular composition of human blood or hemoglobin. Herbivores eat the plants. Omnivores eat the plants and the herbivores. Then everyone dies and goes back into the soil.

You can get nutrition from the sun directly through your skin. When your body is flooded with nutrients, antioxidants, minerals, and vitamins, it naturally protects itself against ultraviolet rays by releasing melatonin. There's also information that comes in through the light spectrum that turns on your hormones and other internal mechanisms that naturally protect you against the environment. Greens are the engine for the closed organic life cycle. Remember to "just eat real food."

Light has a direct effect on our food and health and is a critical part of the closed organic cycle. Fine-tuning your diet is key. You should constantly make sure your body has the best macro ratios of fat, carbs, and protein. You should also identify inflammatory agents like lectins in foods such as soy, grains, corn, legumes, nightshades, and animals that are fed those. Since the esoteric component of nutrition boils down to light, the focus should be on fine-tuning your diet and sourcing the best quality of nutrition. We have established that nutrition comes from light and biophotons. Biophotons are energy that comes from the sun, and then through the closed organic cycle, they're built into plants through chlorophyll. The animals eat the plants, and then we eat the plants or the animals.

Therefore, sunlight is a critical part of nutrition.

Earthing

In the chapter on movement, I talked about incorporating nature into a healthy routine. I don't like treadmills, stair-steppers, and rowing machines and I prefer walking barefoot in the grass. I talked a little about the negative redox potential of the earth and hinted at the health benefits it provides, but here I'd like to expand on that concept.

If the idea of "vibrations" seems "airy-fairy" to you, I encourage you to keep an open mind. We've seen science disregard or dismiss ancient wisdom only to discover these ancient cultures had it right all along.

Many philosophies, especially Eastern philosophies, talk about vibrations and the need to get in tune with nature. And, once again, modern science is just now catching up. New scientific research has begun to identify *cellular seismology* and discovered ways to rapidly identify the different frequencies at which cells vibrate. And these breakthroughs may someday help quantify the exact biomechanical and biochemical responses in the body that drive our health.

But, in the meantime, do your own experimentation. Observe for yourself the results and decide if the impacts on your life are real. Next time you are feeling stressed, take your shoes off and walk in the grass. Within 20 minutes, see if you feel relaxed. I do. Every time. Unquestionably.

But why? Any electrician reading this book will understand the concept of electrical grounding. And practically everyone else should have at least some basic understanding. Living in the United States, you've no doubt noticed that many of your electrical outlets have three openings; two vertical slits that conduct the electricity, and a semi-round hold called the "ground." The purpose of the ground is to protect you from being shocked.

Since this isn't a book on home wiring, I won't go into the specifics, but the short of it is that a ground wire literally goes into the ground at your home. Since the earth has a negative electric charge, and since electricity will follow the path of least resistance, given the opportunity electricity will flow to ground – or into the earth. Lightning rods use the same principle, allowing electricity from lightning to flow harmlessly into the earth rather than electrocuting you.

Earthing is a similar concept. Every second of every day, the cells of your body are interacting with electromagnetic waves from cell phones and electrical wires, from the earth and the sun and the universe itself. But in this modern world, our exposure to man-made electromagnetic waves is a large stressor on our systems. Our cells can become positively charged, changing the natural vibration of our cells, altering our moods, impacting our immune systems, and driving chemical reactions at an atomic level.

Moreover, we tend to wear shoes with rubber soles, travel in automobiles with rubber tires, and insulate ourselves from contact with the earth in this concrete jungle.

Earthing is a simple – and free – way to release negative energy from your body and restore your cells to their natural frequencies. As the great Taoist Master Mantak Chia teaches, the earth has a negative redox potential, which will take out the positively charged toxins and also negative emotions.

Now, of course, all of this advice comes with a few common-sense provisos:

- Make sure the ground you're walking on is safe and free from glass and other debris that can injure you.
- Make sure the grass you walk in isn't sprayed with herbicides, pesticides, and other harmful chemicals.

There is a park in Santa Monica on bluffs overlooking the Pacific Ocean that I go to almost daily. The grass area is several blocks wide and nearly a mile long. I take off my shoes and walk barefoot in the grass in movement meditation. I breathe the fresh air and drink clean, clear water I bring with me. I take nutrition from the sun through my skin, build relationships with some of the regulars in the park, and greet the newcomers with a smile. I connect with nature – literally and figuratively – with my toes in the grass.

Inevitably, I leave the park feeling refreshed and relaxed, and this routine has become a cornerstone for my sleep hygiene. These precious minutes in nature strengthen and fortify my pillars and help alleviate the stress that I come under in my everyday life.

I walk away from the park vibrating at a higher level. My mind is clearer and my emotions are calmed. It is impossible to overstate the importance of this ritual. Some people assume that to be *RippedAt50*, I had to become a gym rat, spending long hours pumping iron. And while it is true that I've grown to enjoy my strength training, it plays a relatively small role in the results I've achieved. I could literally not maintain my physical condition without honoring the 9 Pillars. But my connection to nature is my favorite. I have always truly enjoyed being in nature, and these barefoot strolls are never a chore. They are always a balm for my soul.

Finding Balance

In biology, homeostasis is "the state of steady internal physical and chemical conditions maintained by living systems." Our bodies are engineered to find a perfect balance to perform at an optimum level. In my philosophy, the 9 Pillars need to be balanced for optimum health.

Here, again, is a list of **the 9 Pillars**:

1. The Legacy Pillar
2. The Food Pillar
3. The Rest Pillar
4. The Movement Pillar
5. The Breath Pillar
6. The Thought Pillar
7. The Relationship Pillar
8. The Water Pillar
9. The Nature Pillar

I have also identified stressors that can push the pillars out of alignment. Here, again, are **the 7 Factors of Stress**:

1. Physical Stress
2. Chemical Stress
3. Psychic Stress
4. Nutritional Stress
5. Thermal Stress
6. Electromagnetic Fields (EMF) and Electromagnetic Radiation (EMR) Stress
7. Digital Communications Stress

I believe that, on the whole, the human species is out of balance. In fact, a 2015 study reported that more than 95% of the earth's population is ill—one way or another. Dig deeper and you'll see that the vast majority of disease and illness can be tied directly to the choices we make. Smoking, alcohol, and drug use/abuse are major contributors, but so are our diet and exercise choices. As we discussed in the chapter about sleep, humans are the only animal species who willingly deprive themselves of sleep, and the impact can be dire. Add to that the wholesale changes in agriculture, the explosion of GMOs and glyphosate in our food, the contamination of our air, water, and soil, the pervasive negative impact of media and social media on our emotional wellbeing, and our disconnection with nature, it's no surprise we're suffering from the choices we've made.

Obesity, diabetes, cancer, autoimmune and fertility issues, are just the tip of the iceberg. Our species is in a state of dysbiosis – or imbalance. It seems simple to say, "Just eat real food," but the vast majority of people on this planet don't follow that advice. It breaks my heart to think of children who have only eaten food out of a box or a can; who have never held a real vegetable in their hands, or plucked fresh fruit from a tree.

How did we go so far astray? I have my theories, but I'll save those for another book. I could point fingers at multinational corporations who put their bottom lines above our health. I could describe in detail the nefarious ways they corrupt our food supply and market poison in the guise of "health."

But resentment is toxic and most often self-defeating.

I am grateful for my pain as it teaches me the direction to shift into.

I didn't always eat organic foods. I grew up on an "All-American" diet of cheeseburgers, French fries, and Coca-Cola. I nuked my immune system with antibiotics and willingly robbed myself of sleep. I polluted my body with drugs and alcohol and smoked cigarettes for years. And I suffered the consequences of each of my actions. I paid the price. But I also listened to my pain teacher. I learned – however slowly – the error of my ways. It took me 50 years, but I finally got the 9 Pillars into balance, and my life changed.

And through it all, I learned a deep and abiding respect for nature. We are all-knowing, self-healing creatures of God.

I believe that Mother Nature has provided us with every tool we need to find balance and live optimally. We just need to listen.

In 2005, my personal journey led me to Mexico and Peru. Walking barefoot among the ancient Mayan and Incan temples was a spiritual experience impossible to capture in words. The elders told me that the stones in the temples "remember" the past, and who am I to disagree. I might easily dismiss this as fanciful thinking, but my mind has been opened to so many other seemingly impossible concepts that now the idea doesn't seem strange at all. We're still in the infancy of our human experience, and we've discovered how to store information in crystal and silicon. Couldn't an infinite intelligence devise a universe that stored memories in stone?

All I can tell you is that when my bare skin came into contact with the stones, my mind went easily and almost immediately into a meditative state. Was this real or just some placebo effect? Does it matter?

The point is this: whatever journey you are on – whether you want to lose a few pounds, climb Mt. Everest, or become *RippedAt50*, honor nature in your quest. Mother Nature holds the answers you are looking for. Your job is to listen closely, with an open mind, and follow the good advice she is trying to provide.

In 2006, when I first traveled to the Amazon and experienced ayahuasca, it was virtually unheard of in the United States. Today, ayahuasca ceremonies are conducted nearly every night in Los Angeles, and New York, and San Francisco, and Miami, and other cities across the U.S. and across the world. Sacred tobaccos used in ceremony, from Hapé to Mapacho, were once rare here but are now showing up every-where in the concrete jungle. These are very powerful plants, and they are on the move. My hypothesis is that the jungle is dying, and the long-term viability of these "power plants" is threatened, so the spirits that are bound up in these plants are using man to spread the seeds.

I am a Johnny Appleseed for the 21st century, spreading the seeds of knowledge that I've learned as far and as wide as I can.

I am a humble, kind, and gentle man. My mission is to raise human consciousness and change all systems. My vision is clean air, water, soil, and equitable systems for all mankind...in my lifetime!

Now you have been given a seed. What will you do with it?

As above, so below. This is the natural law of correspondence and the theme of this book. You literally cannot separate your health from the health of the world you live in. Mother Nature is the giver of life and the source of everything that sustains you. Here are some tips to help you build your Nature Pillar:

Bacteria

Remember that your body is made of 10% human cells and 90% bacteria cells. While there are some "bad" bacteria, the vast majority of bacteria inside you are "good" and essential for your health. Honor your microbiome by being a good host and provide the nourishment they need to help you. Think twice about antibiotic use that indiscriminately kills both good and bad bacteria.

The Sun

The sun is the cornerstone of life on earth. It drives our circadian rhythms and provides energy to the plants that feed us, heal us, and produce the oxygen we breathe. The sun also helps regulate our hormones and provides nutrition in the form of biophotonic energy. While it is true that you need to be mindful of the potential harm caused by the sun's rays (especially if you are not regularly exposed to the sun), you need to be more careful about the toxins from sunscreens you rub into your skin! The sun is not to be feared. It is your friend, and you should get out safely into the sunshine and receive the nourishment Mother Nature gives freely.

Earthing

Walking barefoot in the grass is one of the best ways to build your Nature Pillar. Walking is the perfect expression of how your body is meant to move through time and space. The earth has a negative redox potential which will take out the positively charged toxins as well as the negative emotions. Walking barefoot in the grass can be a movement meditation that strengthens your body, relaxes your mind, and grounds your spirit. Do it every day if you can.

Wherever you are in life's journey, Mother Nature holds the answers you are looking for. Listen closely, keep an open mind, and follow the advice she is trying to provide.

And don't mess with the chipmunks.

LOVE

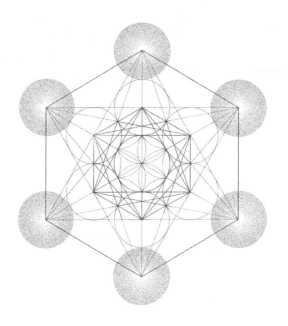

CONCLUSION

"LOVE WINS!!!"

The Ineffable Great Spirit

WRITING A BOOK is a unique experience. This is the first one I've ever written, and it has been an incredible journey. When I set out to write it, I had no idea where it would take me emotionally or spiritually and, as I write this conclusion, I cannot believe what has happened to me in the process.

Uri and I were divorced and separated for a couple of years, but we were still bound to each other in many ways. The children were our major concern, and we did our best to hide the bitterness we still held for each other from them and put the best face on our new situation.

But when we thought the kids were out of earshot, our relationship continued to fester. She was hurt. I was hurt. And we took it out on each other.

"Fuck you."

"No, fuck YOU."

"No. FUCK YOU!"

It seems like no matter what we talked about, that was the subtext of our conversation. And more often than I'd like to admit, that was the actual text of our conversation.

I started dating again, and I know Uri did too. For me, it was a miserable experience. No matter how well I got along with my dates, as soon as we had sex everything changed.

Sex created a sort of quantum entanglement. Suddenly their problems were my problems. Their fears were my fears. Their stresses became my own. I began to resent sex, like it was being used against me. I saw it as some kind of trap.

After a while, I stopped dating at all and became celibate.

I never wanted to get a divorce in the first place. I loved my wife and my family. I didn't want to lose them. But the damage was done. We just had to pick up the pieces and carry on as best we could.

My single prayer was peace and harmony. But still we fought. "Fuck you."

"No, fuck YOU."

"No. FUCK YOU!"

Even when I fell on my face, my prayer remained the same: peace and harmony. By whatever means.

About a year into the divorce, I came out of a psychedelic experience with the realization that I was responsible for my 50% of the relationship. I was still pouring lots of gasoline on the fire and things were burning out of control. In fact, Uri had blocked my calls and texts and did not want to deal with me at all.

How long would it take us to heal from the wounds we were inflicting upon each other. Five years? Ten years? A lifetime? It had to stop.

So I decided that was it. No matter what, I was going to stop pouring my 50% of the gas on the fire. And, believe me, that was hard. But I tried.

Uri noticed the difference, but she was still in fighting mode. I had cut her deep, and she was still reeling in pain.

"Yeah, I noticed the change," she said to me one afternoon. "But you know what?" She paused for dramatic effect. "Don't expect anything from me."

That was a *slightly* nicer way of saying, "Fuck you."

And still, we were connected. We had the kids and they bound us together forever. But the book was also coming along, too.

Uri is a very smart woman and a good businessperson. When I started working on the book, we talked about it. And as bad as our relationship was, Uri wanted me to be successful. The pessimist in me saw this as self-serving. Of course she wanted me to be successful, so I could provide for the kids. But the truth is, it went deeper than that. She wanted Little Troy and Athena to be proud of their father and she truly did want me to be successful.

There are certain things I am good at, and certain things I am not, and Uri knows that. She knew where my Achilles heel was and always protected me. That was one of the things I always loved about her.

Uri had always encouraged me to write a book, and she was happy that I was finally going to give it a go. She helped me. We started to work together on this thing – knowing even then that our divorce would be part of the story. It was scary, but something we both knew needed to be done.

And yeah...it was strange. And familiar. Strangely familiar.

I was spending a lot of time looking backwards then. I was thinking about my childhood, my modeling days, my marriage, and my divorce. What happened? Why? How did these things affect me? How were they still affecting me?

I felt like Uri was living in a shadow of herself. She was so angry. But she was also so afraid. But at this point in our relationship, there was nothing I could say to her. She couldn't hear me.

Many of the problems in our marriage could be traced back to financial fears. We had some lean years, and Uri wanted security. But what she got instead was growing uncertainty. My business had its ups and downs, and the separation only added to our expenses. But more than that, her industry was undergoing massive changes. AI and automation were upending the way things were done, and the future to her looked bleak.

I could relate. I'd lived in a prison of my own making too. But then I'd embraced gratitude and learned to see the world from a different vantage point. Uri and I both drove new cars. We lived in one of the most beautiful places on the planet. We ate organic food and had loving relationships. We had everything we needed. We really didn't have any problems.

But that is not something you can convince someone of. Especially when most of your conversations go like this:

"Fuck you." "No, fuck YOU."

"No. FUCK YOU!"

And still, my single prayer remained the same. Peace and harmony.

Eventually, it was answered. Uri started drinking ayahuasca, and, over time, she made a decision to stop fighting too.

One day, when the kids were at school, she called me over. I thought we were going to have another blowout. But instead she asked me to forgive her.

"Forgive you for what?" I asked.

"The truth is, Troy, I blamed you for everything." "What do you mean," I asked.

"I mean EVERYTHING. When we had money problems, I blamed you. When I had emotional problems, I blamed you. When I was sick, I blamed you. When I didn't have enough energy, I blamed you. In my mind, it was all your fault."

Her eyes filled with tears.

"I'm sorry." She sobbed. And it broke my heart.

Before I knew it, we were holding each other and crying. The dam finally burst, and it overwhelmed us.

And for the next few months, the ice began to melt. We started to talk *to* each other – not *at* each other – for the first time in a long time. And people around us started to notice. "Does this mean you're getting back together?" Dr. Shivambu asked me one day.

"Don't be ridiculous," I scoffed. Being on speaking terms was one thing, but getting back together? Not in a million years would Uri consider it.

But the ice continued to melt. We kept working through our issues and Uri continued drinking the plant medicine.

Soon the first draft of the book was finished, and we were working on the cover design. Uri seemed to have stepped out from her own shadow, and I rediscovered the woman I fell in love with. Could reconciliation even be possible?

Neither of us wanted to allow ourselves to hope for such a thing. The divorce was still fresh in our minds and the wounds we inflicted on each other had not fully healed yet. But, in my heart of hearts, I never wanted to get divorced in the first place.

At about this time I had an offer to go to Rythmia, an all-inclusive, medically licensed luxury resort and retreat center in Costa Rica. They were offering two nights of breath work and four nights of ayahuasca therapy.

It had been seven years since my last experience in 2012. To tell the truth, I am very particular about my sleep, and doing ayahuasca in North America was just not something that appealed to me.

Uri and I had never done an ayahuasca ceremony together. And now she was open to it. The idea was just too exciting for us to pass up.

And so, on October 12, 2019, Uri and I flew to Costa Rica to spend a week at Rythmia.

As excited as I was about the possibility of reconnecting with Uri, I still had serious concerns, too. What was going to happen? Would we just have makeup sex and pretend like none of this ever happened?

I knew we needed to work it through, so I thought we'd spend a lot of time talking about our issues. It's funny, but in my mind, I saw myself sitting in a room with a legal pad, writing everything down, man style.

"So, what are your desires?" I'd ask as I wrote down a bullet-point of her desires. "And your fears?" We'd really make some progress.

But nothing like that actually happened. Thank god! We got there and started doing breath work, and everything fell back into place. We just reconnected. We didn't say anything. We didn't need to.

And then we started doing the plant medicine.

I knew I had to give Uri space for her own mirror gazing, so I dedicated myself to doing the same. How had I failed her as man? As a husband? How could I do better?

Mirror gazing can be a bitch!

Friends had told me I didn't respect women. "What the fuck do you mean?" I'd ask. "C'mon Troy, you know what I mean." "No. Actually I don't. I don't hit women." "I didn't say you did."

"I don't call them bitches." "Not to their faces." "But..."

"But if you can't make money with them or fuck them, you have a habit of dismissing them."

I said that was bullshit and moved on. But was it? Did I disrespect women? Look harder in the mirror. What do you see?

Porn.

When our marriage started breaking up, Uri and I stopped having sex. She cut me off. Worse than that, she cut me off from all physical touch. That made me angry. If adultery can be a crime, then so can that. Cutting someone off emotionally like that is cruel.

Porn was salve on the wound. And then a distraction. And then just background noise?

Looking in the mirror, I knew I could see the darkness it cast on me. Porn had a psychic tug. It shaded my perceptions of women and affected my relationship with my wife. It was objectifying. Ugly.

I had to remove this poison from my life.

And so I have. I am on the NoFap diet. NoFap.com is a website and community that serves as a support community for those who wish to avoid pornography and masturbation.

Ayahuasca ceremonies last a nighttime. They are deep and thorough. The plant medicine does some heavy lifting. When I drink the medicine, I feel like I make 10 years of progress in one night with it.

And Uri and I had already done three nights. It felt like we had made decades of progress already.

The woman I saw in front of me now was not the same one I'd flown down here with. I was seeing her now, not under a shadow, but bathed in tropical light. She was a beautiful flower. Feminine and vital and my heart burst with love when I looked at her.

And so, on the fourth night, before the ceremony started, I asked Uri to marry me. Those eyes, which had once looked at me with such hate and resentment, now filled with tears of joy. She nodded her head and said the one word I most longed to hear: "Yes."

A shaman said he would perform the ceremony at dawn.

The previous three ceremonies had been enlightening. Enjoyable even. This last ceremony was arduous and intense.

The shamans use something called yagé that is a very dense brew of ayahuasca. It is designed to make you purge. It works on your liver, your gall bladder, and your kidneys, and it is powerful stuff.

It's funny. The first time Uri and I got married it was in Vegas. We found this kooky female pastor at one of those drive-through places. I think she was pretty drunk at the time. Anyway, it was a full moon, so I asked if we could have the ceremony outside. I had just returned from Peru where I'd been filming ayahuasca ceremonies. I had the tapes in the trunk of my car, so we asked the Vegas pastor to stop talking and played some footage of a shaman singing an icaro. So, in some ways, our first wedding had something to do with an ayahuasca ceremony too.

But with the second ceremony, Uri and I were kidney deep in it. Before dawn, a male and a female shaman took us outside, where they picked fresh flowers for the ceremony. As the sun came up, they bound our arms together and sang the blessing.

Just then, the first golden rays of the day filtered through the forest and the air danced with life. A chorus of birds and insects lifted their voices in exultation as the shamans elevated our spirits higher with their icaro.

I had crossed the desert and stood now on a higher plane. I had dedicated myself to my wife in a sacred ceremony and stood humbled by the grace the almighty and ineffable spirit had bestowed upon me. But the ayahuasca coursed through me, and I prayed I wouldn't ruin the moment by spilling my guts all over the floor.

On October 18, 2019 Uri and I got married for the second time. And this time, things are going to be different.

It's like I told you at the beginning of this book: Be open to miracles.

LOVE WINS!!!

COVER ART

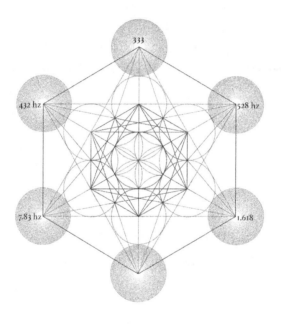

*"No problem can be solved
from the same consciousness that created it."*

Albert Einstein

MY INTENTION FOR writing this book is to elevate consciousness through words. My intention for the cover is to do the same with images. Each individual element of the design has a personal meaning to me. I hope it resonates with you too.

Symbols, like words, have power and magic in them. The great psychologist Carl Jung taught how symbols hold sway over the human mind. We are drawn to symbols in mysterious ways, and there is immense power – and immense danger – in them.

Symbols can be used to enslave as well as to set free.

There are some out there today who use numbers and symbols for black magic. Consumers are compelled to buy products and services that are in not in their best interests, and citizens are enslaved by ideologies not their own. Profits are increased through the use of ancient symbols, and psychological weapons are deployed to illicit ever-stronger emotional reactions that can lead to discord and conflict.

I could have used the pages of this book to rail against the injustices of the world. I might have chosen to point a damning finger at those who poison our bodies and our minds.

Likewise I could have envisioned artwork that reflected the darkness of our world. But I don't want to be *against*. I want to be *for*. For health. For equality. For love.

I am here to set people free, not by selling my own beliefs but by encouraging everyone to open up to their *own* divinity, their *own* creation. I know through my own journey that pathways, no matter how ingrained, can be rewired. I've walked barefoot in the grass and experienced the negative redux potential of the Earth. I've strived to tune myself to Nature's healing frequencies. This knowledge is ancient, but it has remained hidden from us. My mission is to make it freely available to everyone.

I believe that health is the birthright of all people. We are all knowing, self-healing creatures of God. Mother Nature provides us with all the tools we need. She communicates with us through vibrations, but too many have forgotten her language and are cut off from understanding. My book strives to help everyone understand the tools at their disposal. This cover is my attempt to communicate these same thoughts visually.

The cover uses ancient symbols and powerful numbers that have elevated my reality. Whether you understand them or not, their power will work on your mind in mysterious ways. My intention in this section is to explain the significance of the artwork and open your mind to the possibility it represents. By moving these ideas from your subconscious to your conscious mind, I hope to magnify the frequencies they represent so that they may resonate with you more deeply.

Swiss Ball

#RIPPEDAT50 A Journey to Self Love is about finding balance. In it, I teach about the 9 Pillars of Health and describe how my life and my health suffered when certain pillars were neglected and out of balance. Standing on a Swiss ball represents alignment, and shows that vigorous health is possible when the 9 Pillars are aligned. The gray in my beard is there for the world to see, but I wear it with pride! Sure, I've been around the sun 50+ times, but this photograph is a celebration of age, not some idealized representation of my youth. It is also a celebration of a physique I've worked so hard to achieve. Even though I am no spring chicken, I can pick my kids up without pain and feel confident that I am not going to fall and break a hip because of poor stability.

The Swiss ball ramps up the *frequency* of firing in the part of the nervous system that activates the deeper musculature whose primary role is to stabilize the joints including those neurons around the core/abs. The abdominal core starts at the pelvic floor and wraps around the midsection, including the lower back and latissimus dorsi, the hips, hamstrings, and obliques. I am in perfect balance.

Some who know me best, who have heard me rant against corrupt officials and covert operations carried out against our citizens might find it ironic that I am wearing stars and stripes in this shot. But that doesn't mean I am *against* our country. Far from it! I love it, imperfections and all. I am proud to be an American and embrace the positive aspects of the American Dream in the artwork: Life, Liberty, and the Pursuit of Happiness.

Look past the Swiss ball and you'll see numbers and symbols that go beyond six-pack abs. The Natural Law of Correspondence, which states "as above, so below" is represented here. The cover art design is a reminder that there is an art and a science behind optimum health, and is my way of paying homage to the ancient wisdom that has guided me.

Metatron's Cube

This complex geometric shape – comprised of 13 circles with lines extending from the center of each circle to the center of all other circles – represents all shapes in God's creation.

In Greek, meta means "beyond" and tron means the "matrix." Metatron is the name Enoch received after his transformation into an angel, his manifestation beyond the matrix. He is also sometimes equated with Thoth, the Celestial Scribe. He guards the Tree of Life, and presides over the Book of Life, or the Akashic Records. He directly represents our capacity for ascension and our ability to access spiritual power.

All 5 of the Platonic solids can be found in Metatron's Cube. These are the building blocks of life. In the times of Plato, you could be put to death for speaking of them outside the Mystery School. Today it is time for our great awakening. The entire periodic table of elements conforms to an atomic structure based on the Platonic Solids. Modern physics, chemistry, and biology have all begun rediscovering these sacred patterns. The cube has been used as a holy glyph, drawn around an object or person to heal and to ward off demons, or negative energies, and clear them from our lives.

The Divinity Code (333)

333 is a number that speaks to me. It is a number that I have always recognized as *my* number. My birthday numerology boils down to 333. It represents the Father, Son, and the Holy Spirit; the Mind, Body, and Soul. 333 is the Divinity Code.

333 also adds up to 9, which represents the 9 Pillars of Health. 9 is the number of completion. It embodies my mission: to channel and speak my soul's truth using my gifts as a co-creator with the universe. 3 is the number of biological oscillators: brain, heart, and gut. When they are aligned, you have full integrity. For me it's all about full integration without separation. 333 represents connection to the Ineffable Great Spirit.

The Love Frequency (528 Hz)

528 Hz has been called "The Love Frequency" because it resonates at the heart of everything. Bees buzz at 528 Hz. Chlorophyll vibrates at 528 Hz. The King's Chamber in the Great Pyramid resonates at 528 Hz. John Lennon even recorded "Imagine" in 528 Hz. Called the "Miracle" note, "MI" of the original Solfeggio musical scale, researchers have discovered that this frequency was used by ancient healers to perform miracles and produce blessings. In 2010, 528 Hz supposedly was used to clean an area of the BP oil spill in the Gulf of Mexico in just one day.

Phi (1.618)

Like pi, phi is a very special number in math, which is usually rounded to 1.618. It is derived by dividing a line into two parts so that the longer part divided by the smaller part is also equal to the whole length divided by the longer part. It is commonly symbolized using the 21st letter of the Greek alphabet: phi.

The ratio 1.618:1 is known as the Golden Ratio, and recurs in things that are considered beautiful. Mona Lisa exhibits this ratio, as does a pineapple skin, the center of a sunflower, and a spiral galaxy. Each bone in our fingers is phi from the next, and Mecca sits at the phi ratio latitude of Earth.

The Schumann Resonance (7.83 Hz)

7.83 Hz is also known as the Schumann Resonance, or the Earth's Om. It is the frequency at which our planet vibrates. While this sub-sonic frequency is below our hearing range, there is no doubt we feel it. Our organs regulate their processes by it. Our bodies use it as feedback to function optimally. Chances are, you have suffered the ill effects of the absence of this frequency. Because the Schumann Resonance only extends about 30,000 feet above the Earth, and commercial air travel typically takes place between 33,000 and 42,000 feet, you may have felt the effects and called it jetlag.

The Healing Frequency (432 Hz)

In modern music, "A" is commonly tuned to 440 Hz. It has been reported that great musicians such as Mozart and Verdi tuned "A" to 432 Hz. You may think that a difference of 8 vibrations per second is of no consequence, but that is where you are wrong.

Most Modern music is tuned to 440 Hz, which has been observed to cause anxiety. Music recorded at 432 Hz, however, has a soothing effect. What could explain this phenomenon? I believe it is because 432 Hz corresponds with the Schumann Resonance. When the music that reaches our ears vibrates in harmony with the Earth (and all the cells of our body) we naturally feel more in tune with nature.

If you want to overcome anxiety, lower your blood pressure, and decrease your heart rate; relax to the hum of life in the forest, or listen to music by my dear friend, Ralph Smart.

Flower of Life

The Flower of Life has been found in ancient sites around the world. The Book of Genesis in the Bible actually describes the formation of the Seed of Life, or the Genesis Pattern during the 6 days of Creation. After the Seed of Life, the Flower of Life is formed and the Tree of Life (Sefirot, Kabbalah, Yggdrasil) can be found within it. By extending the Flower of Life slightly further, we get the 13 Sphered Fruit of Life. And finally when straight lines (masculine) connect the centers of all 13 circles (feminine), Metatron's Cube is formed.

Final Thoughts

Taken as a whole, these symbols and images represent free energy. If we are to stay in alignment with the Natural Law of Correspondence, we must access the free energy in ourselves and harness it. It is my way of showing that optimum health is within reach; that ascension is attainable. Einstein believed that no problem could be solved from the same level of consciousness that created it. With 95% of people on this planet living with some form of illness, I believe it is self-evident that we need to elevate our consciousness to survive.

I am here to set people free; the Pied Piper of human liberation. The text of my book deals with the ill health effects of discord, dysfunction, and dysbiosis. The cover is meant to represent an aspirational vision of balance and alignment through the natural laws of the universe. The formulae are there for anyone to use. The ancient wisdom is free to all.

It takes a foundation of health to access the higher spiritual realms and stave off self-sabotage. Otherwise you're stuck in your reptilian brain, constantly looping the same reality with the same stale energy. We're evolving. That mind no longer suits us. You can look at the book's cover, the art in the final chapter, or at any other sacred geometry to get activated and elevated. The cover will speak to your soul whether your conscious mind is aware of it or not.

Nature has all the healing frequencies we need. **The Schumann resonance and Solfeggio frequencies can raise our vibration.** Forest bathing, wild water swimming, barefoot grounding, crystal bowl sound healings, hypnotic binaural beats are all healing mechanisms; healing tools. Getting back to nature in all its facets is what I teach. But of course light has dark, yin has yang, and pain can be a great teacher. Being discordant and dysfunctional is all well and good too. The bad will eventually lead us back to balance.

It's all up to YOU.

What do YOU love?
What is YOUR dream?

_____

_____

_____

_____

_____

_____

_____

_____

_____

_____

_____

_____

_____

_____

_____

_____

_____

_____

_____

_____

_____

I am creating...

_____

_____

_____

_____

_____

_____

_____

_____

_____

_____

_____

_____

_____

_____

_____

_____

_____

_____

_____

_____

I am grateful for...

Made in the USA
Coppell, TX
23 June 2024

33850713R00115